Health Education and Promotion

This comprehensive textbook provides students with an accessible overview of both the key concepts and practical skills required to work in the field of health education and promotion.

Primarily aligned with the core competencies identified by the National Health Education Commission, Inc. Areas of Responsibility and designed as ideal preparation for those taking the Certified Health Education Specialist (CHES) examination, this book offers both the theoretical foundations and practical skills required to fulfill a range of roles. From program planning and evaluation to communication and leadership, each chapter details best practices based on the latest research, as well as case studies to show its application in multiple settings. Each chapter is also supported by discussion questions and activities to enable students to engage further with the content.

This is an essential text for students taking a range of courses in health promotion, education, and planning, as well as those preparing for the CHES examination.

Diana Karczmarczyk is a Master Certified Health Education Specialist and holds an MPH degree in Public Health with a focus on community health education and a PhD in Education with a minor in public health and a specialization in international education. She has been teaching public health courses in higher education for almost 20 years on topics including men's health, women's health, sexuality and human behavior, health education and promotion, health behavior theory, program planning and evaluation, personal health and wellness, social determinants of health, and community needs assessments and partnerships.

Sara T. Pappa, a Master Certified Health Education Specialist (MCHES), is an assistant professor and holds a BS in Health Education and Promotion, an MA in Exercise Physiology, and a PhD in Health Education and Promotion. In addition to teaching, she directs a regional falls prevention initiative for older adults. She has extensive experience in managing public health projects at the local, regional, and state levels. Her experience includes implementing and evaluating health promotion programs, conducting community health needs assessments, developing and evaluating community health improvement plans, media outreach, grant writing and administration, coalition development, and strategic planning.

Health Education and Promotion

A Skills-based Approach

Diana Karczmarczyk and Sara T. Pappa

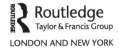

Routledge
Taylor & Francis Group

LONDON AND NEW YORK

Credit line: © Getty Images

First published 2025
by Routledge
4 Park Square, Milton Park, Abingdon, Oxon OX14 4RN

and by Routledge
605 Third Avenue, New York, NY 10158

Routledge is an imprint of the Taylor & Francis Group, an informa business

British Library Cataloguing-in-Publication Data
A catalogue record for this book is available from the British Library

Library of Congress Cataloging-in-Publication Data
Names: Karczmarczyk, Diana, author. | Pappa, Sara, author.
Title: Health education and promotion / Diana Karczmarczyk and Sara T. Pappa.
Description: Abingdon, Oxon; New York, NY: Routledge, 2024. | Includes bibliographical references and index.
Identifiers: LCCN 2024015409 (print) | LCCN 2024015410 (ebook) | ISBN 9781032823973 (hbk) | ISBN 9781032267876 (pbk) | ISBN 9781003504320 (ebk)
Subjects: LCSH: Health education—United States. | Health promotion—United States.
Classification: LCC RA440.5 .K37 2024 (print) | LCC RA440.5 (ebook) |
DDC 362.10973—dc23/eng/20240411
LC record available at https://lccn.loc.gov/2024015409
LC ebook record available at https://lccn.loc.gov/2024015410

ISBN: 978-1-032-82397-3 (hbk)
ISBN: 978-1-032-26787-6 (pbk)
ISBN: 978-1-003-50432-0 (ebk)

DOI: 10.4324/9781003504320

Typeset in Sabon
by codeMantra

I am excited to dedicate this book to our future public health colleagues and collaborators. May the lessons we have shared in this book serve as a guide in your work and prepare you for an amazing career. Thank you in advance for your work and service to communities everywhere.

—Diana Karczmarczyk PhD, MPH, MCHES®

I lovingly dedicate this book to my family, for their unwavering support throughout the writing and editing process. Thank you Gerard, Christina, Joey, Lucy, and George for picking up the slack around the house, meal planning and cooking, and otherwise encouraging me to go the distance – I could not have done this without you!

—Sara T. Pappa PhD, MCHES®

Contents

List of Figures and Tables   ix
List of Authors   xi
Preface   xiii
Acknowledgments   xv

1   Introduction to Health Education and Promotion   1

2   Essential Skills and Competencies: Setting Strong Foundations   23

3   Assessing Communities: Understanding the Needs and Gaps   39

4   Evaluating Programs: Measuring for Success   61

5   Planning and Implementing Interventions and Programs: Engaging Process
    for Impact   79

6   Advocating: Working Toward Change   103

7   Communicating: Sharing Information Effectively   127

8   Leading and Managing: A Role for Everyone   143

9   Professional Development: Strategies for Effectiveness   161

10 Implications for the Future   179

Index   201

Figures and Tables

Figures

2.1	Sample job description	35
3.1	MAPP 2.0 Model	49
3.2	PRECEDE-PROCEED Model	53
4.1	Framework for Program Evaluation in Public Health	70
5.1	Sample Work Plan and Timeline	89
5.2	The Health Impact Pyramid	91
8.1	Sample Meeting Agenda	154
9.1	Bloom's Taxonomy	171
10.1	The 10 Essential Public Health Services	187

Tables

1.1	Definitions of Dimensions of Health	6
1.2	Ottawa Charter Components by Health Promotion Action	11
1.3	Examples of Social Determinants of Health Domains	14
2.1	Eight Areas of Responsibility for CHES® and MCHES®	25
2.2	Comparison of CHES® and MCHES® Examination by Audience, Content, and Job Duties	33
3.1	Limitations for Addressing Health Concerns	44
3.2	MAPP Model Phases	47
3.3	MAPP 2.0 Model Phases	50
3.4	CHANGE Action Steps	52
4.1	Examples of Goals and Objectives	63
4.2	Benefits and Challenges of an Internal versus External Evaluator	65
4.3	Types of Evaluation	67
5.1	Steps in Planning	82
5.2	Sample Mission and Vision Statements	85

5.3   Sample Goal Statements   86
5.4   SMART Objectives   87
5.5   Budget Categories   90
5.6   Levels of Prevention   95
5.7   Main Types of Health Education and Promotion Interventions and Programs   97
5.8   Social-Ecological Model Levels   99
6.1   Components of an Elevator Speech   116
6.2   Phases to Present Proposal to City Council   120
6.3   Examples of Advocacy Evaluation Methods   123
7.1   Key Components in a Successful Health Communication Campaign   129
8.1   Selection of Characteristics of Effective Leaders and Managers   145
8.2   Organizations that Offer Leadership Development Training   155
8.3   Common Language in HES Job Titles   157
9.1   Ten CPH Domains   167
9.2   Examples of Specialized Professional Organizations   175
10.1   Examples of Federal Public Health Agencies   185

Authors

Diana Karczmarczyk PhD, MPH, MCHES®

Dr. Karczmarczyk is a Master Certified Health Education Specialist and holds an MPH with a focus on community health education and a PhD in Education with a minor in public health and a specialization in international education. She has extensive experience in managing and leading public health projects at the local, state, and national levels and has taught public health courses for over 20 years on topics including men's health, women's health, sexuality and human behavior, health education and promotion, health behavior theory, program planning and evaluation, social determinants of health, and community needs assessments and partnerships.

Sara T. Pappa PhD, MCHES®

Affiliation – Marymount University

Dr. Pappa, a Master Certified Health Education Specialist, is an assistant professor and holds a BS in Health Education and Promotion, an MA in Exercise Physiology, and a PhD in Health Education and Promotion. In addition to teaching, she directs a regional falls prevention initiative for older adults. She has extensive experience in managing public health projects at the local, regional, and state levels. Her experience includes implementing and evaluating health promotion programs; conducting community health needs assessments; developing and evaluating community health improvement plans; media outreach; grant writing and administration; coalition development; and strategic planning.

Preface

This idea for this textbook originated at Dr. Pappa's kitchen table. We were brainstorming ways to better prepare future public health colleagues and we decided that, between our collective 50+ years of working in public health and academia, we had a lot we wanted to share. A book made perfect sense!

After many years of teaching experience, we both feel that many textbooks miss opportunities to explore and practice the key skills required to do this important work. Furthermore, we believe that it is not necessary to wait until individuals are employed in this work before learning and using these skills. The reality is that the specific skills that public health professionals have are highly transferable, making them incredibly valuable in any workplace. We wanted to share what we know about public health, and specifically what we know about health education and promotion, and infuse it into the classroom experience for learners.

We want this textbook to be used as a bridge to fill the gaps between the concepts and theory of public health and the practical everyday skills needed to succeed in the field. We included multiple activities for skill-based discussions and opportunities for practice, *Did You Know?* sidebar boxes with information on current health education and promotion topics and resources, and *Concepts in Action* that explore real-world scenarios. Learning objectives, key terms, and web resources are also included in each chapter. The chapter sizes are manageable and will easily fit into a semester course. We also know that the topics covered in each respective chapter could be a semester-long course on their own. Having acknowledged that, we enthusiastically encourage learners to explore the resources we provide to follow and nurture their own curiosities.

Acknowledgments

We want to offer our thanks to the team at Routledge, especially Grace McInnes, Russell George, Evie Lonsdale, and Amy Thomson for your complete support for this project and guiding us through all the stages to publication, even when we hit a few bumps along the way.

A special thanks to Hank, for always being by my side as I drafted content, no matter how long the hours.

—Diana Karczmarczyk PhD, MPH, MCHES®

I want to acknowledge and thank my co-author, Diana, for her steadfast support, guidance, and knowledge throughout this entire process. Her experience with publishing and her kind and patient personality often provided a calming atmosphere in which to write this book. She willingly took on the big lift of making final edits, reference corrections, and formatting of the chapters. I am very grateful to know her both personally and professionally and look forward to our future collaborations.

—Sara T. Pappa PhD, MCHES®

CHAPTER 1

Introduction to Health Education and Promotion

Learning Objectives

After reading this chapter, learners will be able to:

- Explain the roles of health education and promotion professionals in five primary settings
- List key historical events in the health education and health promotion field
- Define four dimensions of health
- Describe how health disparities impact public health outcomes

Keywords

- Dimensions of Health
- Health Disparities
- Health Education Specialist
- Health Equity
- Intersectionality
- Physical Health

- Psychological Health
- Public Health
- Social Determinants of Health
- Social Health
- Spiritual Health
- Tailoring

Self-Reflection Questions

Take a moment and reflect on these questions:

1. What does a health education or health promotion professional actually do?
2. What do you think are the challenges and opportunities for a professional in this field?

DOI: 10.4324/9781003504320-1

The **public health** profession is composed of individuals committed to "promot[ing] and protect[ing] the health of people and the communities where they live, learn, work and play" (American Public Health Association [APHA], 2021b, para. 1). To ensure that the health of individuals and communities is optimal, there are multiple specialties within public health. These specialties include, but are not limited to, health policy, epidemiology, environmental health, health education, and health promotion. Public health professionals within these specialties work together to promote and protect the health of populations across a wide variety of settings.

Professional preparation for each of these specialties can vary from the academic degrees that are required to the certifications that professionals are encouraged to complete and maintain throughout their careers. For example, public health professionals may pursue certification as a Certified Health Education Specialist (CHES®). This certification has a distinct process for obtaining the initial certification and completing the required continuing education to maintain the credentials. This national certification enables employers to hire individuals with specific proven competencies in health education and health promotion. In 2023, more than 450 employers in the United States recognized and preferred hiring HES with a CHES® or MCHES® certification (National Commission for Health Education Credentialing, Inc. [NCHEC], n.d.-a).

Certified Health Education Specialist

The CHES® certification is further explored in Chapter 2, with specific information on the qualifications for the credential, the expected competencies, and details about the exam.

While each public health professional works toward improving health outcomes, those who plan, develop, and implement health education and health promotion programs provide a key element of supporting positive health behaviors. The successful and effective delivery of these programs does not happen by chance. They are the result of planned, consciously constructed learning opportunities with the goal of improving health and health outcomes. Health education and promotion professionals are often referred to as **Health Education Specialists**. This chapter will review significant events in the field of health education and promotion and how these have shaped the role and responsibilities of HES in today's workforce.

Terminology in This Book

The acronym HES is used in this book to refer to Health Education Specialists, health promotion professionals, community health specialists, and community health educators to be inclusive of each of these roles.

Health Education and Promotion Professionals

The U.S. Bureau of Labor Statistics (BLS) describes HES as individuals "who [teach] people about behaviors that promote wellness. They develop strategies to improve the well-being of individuals and communities" (2022, What They Do, para. 1).

The essential skills and competencies needed by HES to successfully support the well-being of the communities and ensure that health education and promotion programs happen consistently and appropriately include assessing communities, planning programs, implementing programs, evaluating programs, advocating, communicating, leading and managing, and professional development. In addition to the job duties of a HES being highly varied, they are also dependent upon work location.

> ### Skills and Competencies Framework
>
> The skills and competencies needed by HES are further introduced in Chapter 2 and explored in subsequent chapters throughout this book. Multiple examples are provided in each chapter from urban, rural, and suburban settings across the United States to highlight how these skills and competencies make an impact on the specific audiences and communities where HES work.

Primary Settings

The five primary settings for HES include public health departments, worksites, hospitals or healthcare organizations, nonprofits, and educational institutions (U.S. Bureau of Labor Statistics [BLS], 2022, What They Do, para. 4–8). In local, state, and national health departments, HES may create and implement public health campaigns on a wide range of health topics. These might include control of TB, emergency preparedness, immunizations, physical activity, tobacco use, or proper nutrition. For example, as part of the response to COVID-19, many local health departments took on the task of providing mass vaccination clinics. HES may develop educational materials for use in the community and by public health officials. They may also collaborate with local, regional, state, and national colleagues on campaigns or coalitions. They may also apply for grants, offer grants, and implement grant-funded programs designed to improve and protect the public's health.

At worksites, HES may create programs designed to improve the health and wellness of employees. For example, they may develop incentives for employees to adopt healthy behaviors, such as reduced health insurance premiums for managing high blood pressure, or recommend changes in the workplace to improve employee health, such as an on-site fitness center and classes. Employee wellness programs are becoming a common employee benefit as more employers are recognizing their role in promoting health and well-being. HES may also work for an organization's training department and teach courses on health-related topics specific to the job for the employees or the people that they interact with.

In hospitals and other healthcare organizations, HES may work individually with patients, their families and caregivers, and medical providers. They may implement interventions or programs designed to educate about health status, disease management, and treatment options. For example, they may offer education sessions to medical providers on health behavior coaching techniques or lead a session on stress management. They may serve as a connection to the larger community by contributing to population health efforts, including community health needs assessments and subsequent community health improvement plans.

In nonprofit organizations, specifically those that are health-related, HES may develop and implement programs and create materials about specific health issues for diverse audiences. They may identify funding opportunities, write grants, and coordinate fundraisers to sustain the work of the nonprofit and create new programs and services. For example, they may find a corporate grant to expand upon an existing program at the organization and submit an application. HES may also advocate for programs and policies by reaching out to and educating elected local, state, and federal officials.

HES may also have a primary role in education and training. While this may include teaching in elementary and secondary school grades, this may also include teaching at a police or fire academy to prepare first responders with stress management techniques. HES may develop a curriculum for a community college or four-year institution as a full-time or part-time faculty member. Courses may be focused on health topics such as community health, chronic disease management, or infectious disease, and these courses might also be designed to prepare future HES and public health professionals for the workforce.

Activity 1.1: Discussion

Visit the U.S. Bureau of Labor Statistics and read about what a HES does at healthcare facilities, nonprofit agencies, public health departments, and schools at https://www.bls.gov/ooh/community-and-social-service/health-educators.htm#tab-2

Compare and contrast the duties of HES and discuss your responses to the following questions:

1. How are the duties similar?
2. How are the duties different?
3. What skills are required for each type of role?

Current Workforce and Projections

There were approximately 59,600 HES employed in 2021, with the government (26%) as the largest employer (BLS, 2022, Work Environment, para. 2). The expected job growth for HES is projected to be 12%, with an average of 16,000 jobs available each year mostly to fill vacancies left by those retiring from the workforce (BLS, 2022, Job Outlook, para. 1–2).

Current Workforce

Challenges and opportunities for the current public health and health education and promotion workforce are further explored in Chapter 10.

HES will continue to be called upon to develop and implement programs and interventions that promote healthy behaviors as chronic diseases remain the leading causes of death in the United States (Centers for Disease Control and Prevention [CDC], 2022). Professionals who understand health behaviors and can develop effective responses to them as part of the public health and medical system are critical (APHA, 2015). In addition, the COVID-19 pandemic reemphasized the continued need for a well-trained public health workforce, of which HES are a vital component. Finally, the need to improve the overall quality and outcomes of healthcare is important as governments, healthcare providers, and social service providers work to reduce healthcare costs (APHA, 2015; BLS, 2022, Job Outlook). Educating people about how to prevent and manage chronic diseases will help to improve quality of life, as well as reduce healthcare costs. Each of these factors will continue to play important roles as the demand for HES grows.

Health Dimensions

There are many definitions of health; however, the one that is generally accepted as the leading definition for public health efforts is from the World Health Organization (WHO). WHO defines health as "a state of complete physical, mental and social well-being and not merely the absence of disease or infirmity" (World Health Organization [WHO], 2022, para. 1). This definition was included in the constitution of the organization when it was developed in 1948 to "[connect] nations, partners and people to promote health, keep the world safe and serve the vulnerable – so everyone, everywhere can attain the highest level of health" (WHO, 2023a, para. 2). Since its adoption, there has been criticism of the definition. For example, Huber (2011) argues that the definition "minimizes [sic] the role of the human capacity to cope autonomously with life's ever changing physical, emotional, and social challenges and to function with fulfillment and a feeling of wellbeing with a chronic disease or disability" (p. 236). According to the CDC (2023), 60% of adults have at least chronic health condition, such as diabetes or heart disease. In addition, Jadad and O'Grady (2008) argue that:

> Health is not a fixed entity. It varies for every individual, depending on their circumstances. Health is defined not by the doctor, but by the person, according to his or her functional needs. The role of the doctor is to help the individual adapt to their unique prevailing conditions.
>
> *(p. 781)*

Despite the criticism, this is still the most commonly cited definition of health, and the components of the definition support other key definitions. Specifically, the various aspects of health included in the WHO definition of physical, mental, and social well-being are now commonly referred to as **dimensions of health**. There are multiple health models that depict health dimensions. Bill Hettler, MD, is credited with developing the first wellness model in 1976 with six dimensions of health while he worked as a college health administrator and medical provider at the University of Wisconsin Stevens Point and later went on to establish the National Wellness Institute (Rozen, 2022). Since then, multiple versions and depictions of wellness models with varying health dimensions have been developed over the years. While some models have as many as 15 dimensions, most models include physical, spiritual, social, and psychological as the primary health dimensions, as indicated in Table 1.1.

Table 1.1 Definitions of Dimensions of Health

Dimension	Definition
Physical health	Generally refers to an individual's ability to complete activities for daily living
Spiritual health	Generally refers to an individual's sense of purpose in life and their ability to practice gratitude
Social health	Generally refers to an individual's connections with others
Psychological health	Generally refers to an individual's ability to cope or manage with stressful situations

Physical health can include general tasks such as getting ready for the day and carrying out your daily responsibilities. Physical health can also include things that may not be visible, such as an individual's cholesterol and blood glucose levels. If these are not at recommended levels, health issues such as a heart attack or diabetes could result. **Spiritual health** is often associated with religion, though it is not a requirement for finding meaning and purpose in life. Feeling connected to one's community and being in nature can be ways to strengthen spiritual health. **Social health** is not necessarily about the quantity of relationships, rather it is about the quality of a relationship or relationships in a person's life. Being able to communicate vulnerable emotions with someone as part of a support system can positively impact health outcomes. In response to the growing public health concern of loneliness and isolation, the Office of the U.S. Surgeon General released *Our Epidemic of Loneliness and Isolation* in 2023 to call attention to the importance of social connection and the role of belonging in overall well-being (U.S. Office of the Surgeon General, 2023). Finally, **psychological health** is often listed as mental or emotional health in wellness models. Though the description remains consistent. Psychological health describes a person's ability to navigate through stressful situations. Individuals may experience short-term and acute stressful moments, such as being called in to speak with a supervisor at work, or long-term stress, such as a diagnosis of a chronic health issue that requires regular interventions. Psychological health may benefit from a focus on developing effective stress management skills, coping strategies, and enhancing resiliency.

It is important to remember that these dimensions "can be thought of as existing on a continuum" for individuals across their lifespan (Milstein & Karczmarczyk, 2021, p. 1). Optimal health can be described as a point at which an individual has achieved their highest level of wellness in any of the dimensions. There may be times when one dimension of health is optimal for an individual, and other dimensions may not be. Optimal health perspectives also vary. For example, while a person who has lost a limb may not be able to perform a physical activity at the same speed or for as long as someone without a limb loss, each of these individuals can achieve their own level of optimal physical health. Public health is an incredibly optimistic field in that sense. The point is to celebrate the achievements of individuals and see how they have improved in their muscle strength, endurance, and heart health for instance, as opposed to simply weight loss. While achieving optimal wellness may be a goal for many, achieving and maintaining healthy behaviors can be challenging, as it may require constant and ongoing efforts. HES are uniquely equipped with skills and knowledge so that they are able to not only appreciate the difficulty in trying to change a habit or behavior but also identify opportunities to improve policies, create programs, or offer education aimed at eradicating those that hinder health and promote those that improve and foster positive health. HES are equipped with an understanding of human behavior and health behavior theories.

Significant Historical Events

Examples of the delivery of health education to individuals and communities can be found throughout history. Typically, messages about health have been provided by those with medical training, such as physicians, nurses, and midwives. For example, between 1925 and the 1960s, nurse midwives were credited for their role in developing and disseminating childbirth education and promoting breastfeeding (Rooks, 2022). However, early health educators also included religious leaders. For example, in addition to moral instruction priests played a significant role in delivering health education in the Middle Ages (Temkin, 1940). The evolution of what has been promoted as healthy and how it has been promoted is also fascinating. Understanding the evolution of the profession is important because this aids in preparing HES to perform their duties and provides context for the challenges that remain in the field.

> ### SIDEBAR: DID YOU KNOW?
>
> Health behavior theories are the foundation of understanding, explaining, and predicting health behaviors. Undergraduate and graduate programs in health promotion typically offer at least one course to review several of the most commonly used theories and models used to inform the development of programs and interventions to improve health outcomes.
>
> To learn more about health behavior theories, please visit https://cancercontrol.cancer.gov/sites/default/files/2020-06/theory.pdf to review *Theory at a Glance* (Rimer & Glanz, 2005). This is a free publication that summarizes key concepts of eight theories that HES can use in their roles.

Historical Review

The following section summarizes significant events in the history of health education and promotion primarily in the 20th century and beyond. It is not intended to serve as a complete review of historical events.

Ancient Civilizations

Ancient Greek physicians provided health information to individuals, regardless of profession or economic status (Temkin, 1940). However, Dr. Temkin, a renowned medical historian, references an evolution in their practice when differentiated guidance was provided by "Hippocratic authors as well as in Diocles of Carystus, the great physician of the 4th century B.C." because it was recognized that there were those who were able to "devote their time to following all the minute prescriptions of the Greek physicians" compared with those who couldn't due to work responsibilities (p. 1092). Therefore, differentiation in messaging occurred that resonated with different members of the community. This may have been an early example of tailoring health information. **Tailoring** describes the practice of providing specific information and guidance to an audience with their specific needs and the context of those needs in mind. So, creating different health promotion messages and recommendations for those with limited time may have a higher likelihood of being adopted.

Overall, physicians were primarily promoting guidance for maintaining and promoting health with specific foods to eat and avoid, exercises to perform, and sleep behaviors to maintain (Temkin, 1940). However, these texts were often written in Greek, not Latin, which limited the information to the select Romans who could read Greek (Temkin, 1940). This limitation essentially created health inequities for the majority of individuals. **Health inequities** are considered to be unfair or stemming from some form of injustice (National Heart, Lung, and Blood Institute, 2019). The topics of health equity and **health disparity**, the differences in health outcomes as a result of these inequities, are explored later in the chapter though it is vital to highlight here that challenges in health equity were documented (and later identified as such) for centuries.

Between 1450 and 1500, multiple examples of text written in German and French, likely by physicians and surgeons, are cited as early examples of mass distribution of health education for potentially the community at large given its use of poetic language (Temkin, 1940). According to Temkin, the information outlined guidance on pregnancy and child development, including diet and bathing (1940).

These early examples of health education demonstrate many components of contemporary health education and promotion efforts highlighting how long-standing the practice truly is. However, it was not until the 20th century that the academic preparation and credentials of health education and promotion professionals were formalized and expanded beyond medical professionals.

20th Century: Academic Preparation of Health Professionals

In 2003, the Institute of Medicine [now known as the National Academy of Medicine] Committee on Educating Public Health Professionals for the 21st Century (IOMCEPHP) released *Who Will Keep the Public Healthy? Educating Public Health Professionals for the 21st Century*. This publication outlines the origins and evolution of academic preparation for public health professionals in the United States.

In the early 1900s, Wickliffe Rose, Founder of the Rockefeller Sanitary Commission, wanted to address the lack of an educational pathway to develop public health professionals "...who would devote their entire careers to controlling disease and promoting health at a population level" and enlisted Abraham Flexner to help (Institute of Medicine Committee on Educating Public Health Professionals [IOMCEPHP], 2003, p. 42). In October 1914, Flexner convened 11 public health representatives and 9 trustees from the Rockefeller Sanitary Commission to identify the various roles within public health. The group agreed on three main categories: (1) those with executive authority to include local and state health officials, (2) subject matter experts such as infectious disease experts, and (3) those that supported local efforts such as public health nurses and safety inspectors (IOMCEPHP, 2003). Rose used this guidance to identify the vision for a university curriculum to ensure that public health professionals would be adequately prepared to serve in these roles. Rose's original vision included academic programs at universities across the country, separate from medical schools, with a focus on health education and skill building with field-based practice opportunities (IOMCEPHP, 2003). Interestingly, the first iterations of this vision emphasized the biomedical side of public health and excluded the social and economic context of the work, with "no attention was given to the political sciences or to the need to plan for social or economic reforms" (IOMCEPHP, 2003, p. 42). This meant that the initial curriculums did not include health education, field training, or public health program planning and evaluation that Rose had envisioned. In 1918, the Johns Hopkins University School of Hygiene and Public Health, the first endowed school of public health, opened. According to IOMCEPHP, schools in Boston and Toronto followed, and each of these early schools of public health were well funded, some by the Rockefeller Foundation, and graduated a select number of students (2003). Typically, the students each had a prior medical degree. Therefore, these schools did not meet the vision of training large cadres of future public health professionals in the three categories originally envisioned by Rose (IOMCEPHP, 2003).

A boost to enrollment happened because of a benefit from the passage of the Social Security Act of 1935. It provided federal assistance to states to secure training for public health professionals (Social Security Online, n.d.). As the demand for trained public health educators from local health departments to train higher volumes of public health professionals grew, more specialized training was developed. There was an increase in the number of schools that offered degrees in public health and short-duration training programs lasting a few weeks to a few months were developed across the country to quickly train public health professionals (IOMCEPHP, 2003). According to IOMCEPHP, the 1930s were "prime years of community-based public health education" (2003, p. 44).

In response to the rapid growth and demand for public health education professionals, the Association of Schools of Public Health (ASPH) was formed in 1941 to promote and improve graduate education for public health professionals (IOMCEPHP, 2003). By the 1950s, the consensus was that schools of public health that were accredited were effectively preparing students to enter the profession. However, the main challenges included adequate funding to pay faculty, purchase needed supplies, and expand classroom space for increased enrollments. According to IOMCEPHP (2003), it was during this time that a change occurred that still has implications to date. Schools of public health were competing against medical schools and community hospitals for funding. This meant that to be competitive, faculty needed to turn more toward research and less toward community-based and field training to maintain their public health programs. Over the years, the volume of students in schools of public health has correlated with federal support for grants to support projects and curriculum development (IOMCEPHP, 2003).

20th Century: Public Health Context

While schools of public health were being developed and preparing public health professionals, there were multiple prominent health issues facing Americans. A significant one was tobacco. Between the 1930s and the 1950s, it was common for medical providers to promote tobacco products to patients for stress management in magazines, newspaper advertisements, and directly to patients in their offices (Yale University Library, 2003). While this may seem shocking today given what is known about the health risks associated with smoking, it took advocates years to bring about change. By 1964, the U.S. Surgeon General released *Smoking and Health: Report of the Advisory Committee to the Surgeon General*, which reported that cigarette smoking was "responsible for a 70 percent increase in the mortality rate of smokers over non-smokers" (National Library of Medicine, n.d., para. 5). Cigarette advertisements were banned from television and radio stations regulated by FCC in 1970, with the last ad appearing on January 1, 1971 (History.com, 2009; Truth Initiative, 2017). In 1998, the Master Settlement Agreement (MSA) was signed between the four largest companies and 52 state and territory attorney generals to "settle dozens of state lawsuits brought to recover billions of dollars in health care costs associated with treating smoking-related illnesses" (National Association of Attorney Generals [NAAG], 2023, para. 1). The MSA, an agreement that lasts in perpetuity as long as tobacco companies that were included in the agreement sell cigarettes in the United States, further restricted tobacco advertisements – especially targeting youth (NAAG, 2023). Annual payments from tobacco companies included in the MSA have been used to develop smoking prevention and cessation programs or fund other health improvement efforts.

SIDEBAR: DID YOU KNOW?

Using popular channels to promote health products directly to consumers remains a common strategy. Ads for prescription medication on television, radio, magazines, newspapers, and the internet aimed at consumers, referred to as direct-to-consumer pharmaceutical advertising (DTCPA), rose by 30% between 2013 and 2015 for a total amount of at least $4.5 billion (American Medical Association [AMA], 2015). In 2015, the American Medical Association adopted a policy to demonstrate collective support for a ban on these kinds of advertisements due to the role they play in driving up costs for prescription medications (AMA, 2015). Congress approval would be needed for a DTCPA ban.

Ottawa Charter

A significant event occurred in 1986 that set the foundation for health education and promotion work on a global scale. The first international conference on health promotion met in Ottawa, Canada, and resulted in a charter with goals for health outcomes to be achieved by the year 2000 and beyond (WHO, 2009). Two hundred conference participants from 38 countries collectively pledged to six commitment statements outlined in Table 1.2 (WHO, 2012). These commitments span across policy development, personal development, and changing the healthcare systems to improve health outcomes. These actions were identified at the conference as specific steps for health promotion professionals to engage in to promote and advance health. The sixth commitment did not have a specific action step outlined, though it captures the need for an overall investment in public health as part of a sustainable and scale-able global effort.

SIDEBAR: DID YOU KNOW?

Unnatural Causes: Is inequality making us sick? is a four-hour PBS documentary series that explores the root causes of socioeconomic and racial health disparities. This popular series offers "startling new findings that suggest there is much more to our health than bad habits, health care, or unlucky genes" (California Newsreel, 2008, para. 2).

To learn more about the documentary, please visit https://unnaturalcauses.org/.

Table 1.2 Ottawa Charter Components by Health Promotion Action

Health Promotion Action Type	Commitment of Participants
Build healthy public policy	To move into the arena of healthy public policy and to advocate a clear political commitment to health and equity in all sectors
Create supportive environments	To counteract the pressures toward harmful products, resource depletion, unhealthy living conditions and environments, and bad nutrition; and to focus attention on public health issues such as pollution, occupational hazards, housing, and settlements
Strengthen community action	To respond to the health gap within and between societies and to tackle the inequities in health produced by the rules and practices of these societies
Develop personal skills	To acknowledge people as the main health resource; to support and enable them to keep themselves, their families, and friends healthy through financial and other means; and to accept the community as the essential voice in matters of its health, living conditions, and well-being
Reorient health services	To reorient health services and their resources toward the promotion of health and to share power with other sectors, other disciplines, and, most importantly, with people themselves
	To recognize health and its maintenance as a major social investment and challenges and to address the overall ecological issue of our ways of living

Note: Adapted from "The Ottawa Charter for Health Promotion" by WHO, 2009, pp. 4–5. Retrieved from https://oot.enhance-fcn.eu/pluginfile.php/8077/mod_resource/content/1/WHO_milestones_in_health_promotion.pdf.

Healthy People 1990 and 2000

In the 1979 Surgeon General's report, *Healthy People: The Surgeon General's Report on Health Promotion and Disease Prevention*, the concept of Healthy People was established. The report "...called for a renewed commitment to disease prevention and emphasized the role of both population and community health and individual and personal lifestyle choices and risk factors" (Ochiai et al., 2021, para. 5). By the following year, the U.S. Department of Health and Human Services (HHS) released the first set of Healthy People targets based on existing scientific evidence to be completed within a decade (Ochiai et al., 2021). The goal by 1990 was to "[focus] on health across the life span: the initiative sought to decrease mortality in infants, children, adolescents, and adults, and increase independence among older adults" (Ochiai et al., 2021, para. 7). By 2000, the goal of increasing access to preventive services and reducing health disparities was added, marking the first time the term health disparities was included in Healthy People (Ochiai et al., 2021).

SIDEBAR: DID YOU KNOW?

By 1990, the health education profession took a major leap forward when the Certified Health Education Specialist (CHES®) national certification was first administered (NCHEC, n.d.-b). This credential, along with the more recent Master Certified Health Education Specialist (MCHES®), elevated the profession by recognizing the need to formalize levels of competence in the practice of health education with a certification.

> **National Certification**
>
> More details are provided in Chapter 2 about the progress to date on certifying HES and the evolution of the certification process.

Health Disparities

By 2003, the landmark book *Unequal Treatment: Confronting Racial and Ethnic Disparities in Health Care* was released. The book explores the experiences of persons of color in the healthcare system and the quality of care that they receive to demonstrate the role of race and ethnicity in these settings (Institute of Medicine [IOM], 2003). The abstract of the book stated,

> Racial and ethnic minorities tend to receive a lower quality of healthcare than non-minorities, even when access-related factors, such as patients' insurance status and income, are controlled. The sources of these disparities are complex, are rooted in historic and contemporary inequities, and involve many participants at several levels, including health systems, their administrative and bureaucratic processes, utilization managers, healthcare professionals, and patients.
>
> *(p. 1)*

The authors included recommendations to address and eliminate differences in care such as the availability of translation services, cross-cultural training for medical providers, and data collection on patients to further review practices and assess the impact of interventions (IOM, 2003). Despite the attention that the book received, 20 years since its release there is wide criticism for how little has been done to change the landscape of healthcare to address these disparities. According to Blanding (2022), "the gap between white people and racial and ethnic minorities has remained frustratingly persistent, with little concrete progress to show for the efforts that have been made to close it" (para. 11). Some progress has been made on "improving monitoring and performance measurement on racial metrics" to help identify opportunities for action and "[m]any health care systems in the United States now do at least some form of implicit bias training for their staff" (Blanding, 2022, para. 12). However, challenges in implementing changes using programs with unsustainable funding has been difficult (Blanding, 2022). Early indications of the implications of the Affordable Care Act also indicate that while it reduced racial and ethnic disparities in health insurance coverage, substantial disparities remain (Buchmueller et al., 2016). The Affordable Care Act is reviewed later in the chapter.

> **Activity 1.2: Discussion**
>
> The Merriam-Webster's definition of racism is "the systemic oppression of a racial group to the social, economic, and political advantage of another" (n.d., Definition 2). In early 2021, Rochelle Walensky, the CDC Director at that time, declared racism to be a serious public health threat (CDC, 2021a). Later that year, multiple cities and counties made similar declarations (APHA, 2021a).

1. Why is it important to declare racism as a serious public health threat?
2. Describe how racism impacts health outcomes.
3. How can HES address and eliminate health disparities to achieve health equity?

To learn more, read the statement made by Director Walensky at https://www.cdc.gov/media/releases/2021/s0408-racism-health.html.

Note: Since the statement was released, the Racism and Health portal was moved to https://www.cdc.gov/minorityhealth/racism-disparities/.

The Evolution of Healthy People

Since its inception, Healthy People has undergone many updates and improvements. Healthy People 2030 focuses on and defines health disparities as "a particular type of health difference that is closely linked with social, economic, and/or environmental disadvantage" (Office of Disease Prevention and Health Promotion [ODPHP], n.d.-a, para. 7). Furthermore, Healthy People 2030 explains that

> Health disparities adversely affect groups of people who have systematically experienced greater obstacles to health based on their racial or ethnic group; religion; socioeconomic status; gender; age; mental health; cognitive, sensory, or physical disability; sexual orientation or gender identity; geographic location; or other characteristics historically linked to discrimination or exclusion.
>
> *(ODPHP, n.d.-a, para. 7)*

With a focus on eliminating health disparities, the Healthy People 2030 framework includes the goal of achieving health equity. Healthy People 2030 defines health equity as "the attainment of the highest level of health for all people" (ODPHP, n.d.-a, para. 6). In order to achieve health equity, it "requires valuing everyone equally with focused and ongoing societal efforts to address avoidable inequalities, historical and contemporary injustices, and the elimination of health and health care disparities" (ODPHP, n.d.-a, para. 6). Including these definitions in Healthy People 2030 is important because it signifies a collective commitment to these efforts and guides those working at the local level with a common language.

Social Determinants of Health

Health status is impacted by a number of factors, including social determinants of health. The CDC defines **Social Determinants of Health** (SDOH) as the "… conditions in the places where people live, learn, work, and play that affect a wide range of health and quality-of-life-risks and outcomes" (2021b, para. 1). According to WHO, SDOH may be more important in influencing health outcomes than health care or individual behaviors accounting "for between 30–55% of health outcomes" (2023b, Overview, para. 5). SDOH conditions have been categorized into five domains. These include (1) Healthcare Access and Quality, (2) Education Access and Quality, (3) Social and Community Context, (4) Economic Stability, and (5) Neighborhood and Built

Environment (ODPHP, n.d.-b). The Health Access and Quality domain describes not just being able to see a provider for a health condition, but having access to high-quality healthcare that ensures the best outcomes for the patient regardless of their background. It also includes access to affordable health insurance. Access to affordable health insurance was a key feature of the Affordable Care Act, also known as the Patient Protection and Affordable Care Act, passed in March 2010 (U.S. Department of Health and Human Services [HHS], 2022). In 2000, the Office on Minority Health released the first ever Culturally and Linguistically Appropriate Services (CLAS) standards for healthcare providers and healthcare organizations to "to advance health equity, improve quality, and help eliminate health care disparities" (Office of Minority Health, n.d., para. 1). The standards address needs such as health literacy and cultural practices to ensure that patient needs are addressed appropriately. Access to quality early childhood education is the focus of the Education Access and Quality domain (Table 1.3).

The impact of SDOH has been well documented in terms of how they impact health disparities and health

> ## SIDEBAR: DID YOU KNOW?
>
> The 2008 report from the Commission on Social Determinants of Health called attention to the variance in life expectancy based on where individuals live. For example, the life expectancy is 80 years in Sweden and Japan, but as low as 50 years in several African countries (CSDH, 2008). The authors explained that across the globe, "at all levels of income, health and illness follow a social gradient: the lower the socioeconomic position, the worse the health" (CSDH, 2008, p. 2). Furthermore, the authors explain health inequity as "systematic differences in health [that] are judged to be avoidable by reasonable action … are, quite simply, unfair" (CSDH, 2008, p. 2). The authors demand a global response to this social justice issue with the three overarching recommendations in a 256-page report. To learn more about the recommendations, please visit https://www.who.int/publications/i/item/9789241563703.

Table 1.3 Examples of Social Determinants of Health Domains

SDOH Domain	Examples
Healthcare access and quality	Access to high-quality healthcare, affordable health insurance, and culturally and linguistically appropriate services
Education access and quality	Access to high-quality early childhood education, high school graduation rates, and affordable higher education
Social and community context	Community and worksite cohesion, participation in elections, discrimination, and justice systems
Economic stability	Poverty, food security, and housing stability
Neighborhood and built environment	Water and air quality, transportation, housing quality, crime, and violence

Note: Adapted from "What are Social Determinants of Health" by Healthy People 2030, US Department of Health and Human Services, Office of Disease.
Prevention and Health Promotion., n.d.-b, para. 1. Retrieved from https://health.gov/healthypeople/priority-areas/social-determinants-health.

outcomes. In 2008, the WHO Commission on Social Determinants of Health released a groundbreaking report acknowledging disparities in health outcomes with three key recommendations to close the gap in a generation (Commission on Social Determinants of Health [CSDH], 2008). The recommendations included improving the living conditions for individuals across their lifespan; remedying the unequal distribution of power, money, and resources; implementing strategies to measure health inequities; developing appropriate interventions; and evaluating the interventions for effectiveness (CSDH, 2008).

The impact was most recently highlighted during the COVID-19 pandemic (Abrams & Szefler, 2020). For example, poverty prevented individuals from accessing testing and treatment; school closings disrupted the ability for millions of school children to access healthy lunches; and, employees who did not have the ability to work from home lost wages and were potentially exposed to the virus during public transit commutes and on-site work days. Overcrowding and homelessness contributed to increased exposure for those with limited financial and/or housing stability. These challenges compounded for individuals making it difficult to focus on health needs while also

---

Concept in Action

Each chapter will also include *Concepts in Action*. These will feature case studies with fictional characters throughout the book to highlight each of the four common work settings to highlight practical examples in the workplace and skills needed. The characters will include Tasha, Sam, José, and Aisha.

Concept in Action 1.1

Background: Sam (they/them) has worked at a local nonprofit as a health programs coordinator for the past three years. They have a Bachelor's degree in Health Education and Promotion. Sam's primary role is to develop educational content and health promotion programs for local communities within the region, with the support of a volunteer Board.

Recently, the Board decided that they wanted to do more innovative programs to support community members. The Board wanted to do something meaningful but didn't know what or how they could help. They ended the meeting by encouraging everyone to brainstorm ideas on how to improve health in the region.

About a week later, Sam was approached by a member of the Board about exploring the Produce Prescription Program that has been incredibly successful in Ohio to provide prescriptions to community members which served as vouchers for free food at a local farmer's market (Prevention Research Center for Healthy Neighborhoods, 2020). Sam reviewed the following website to learn more about the program and watched the brief video linked on the website at http://prchn.org/prx/.

A few days later, the member of the volunteer Board called Sam and asked, "So, what do you think? Can we make this happen here or what? I think it would get us a lot of media attention and we could make a real difference. We could start in our city and go from there." Sam paused before responding. "Here is the thing, this is a wonderful program. It really is. I can see why it worked for these cities. But before we consider if this could work here, we have to stop and think about our own communities that we serve and their needs." Sam paused again, waiting for a response. "I don't understand why we wouldn't do that program here, Sam. I think our city would be a great place to pilot this and try it out. It seems easy enough. Ok, so I know that we don't have a farmer's market every week, but we could make those happen. And, we don't have an amazing pharmacist here to identify and refer patients, but we could find one. How hard could it be? I would guess that my neighbors would want to get some free food. I mean, as long as we just hand them the voucher they will show up. Right? So, why not?" The volunteer sounded hopeful, but was also starting to realize how much work is involved in developing even a pilot program.

Sam replied, "I really appreciate your energy on this. They do make it look easy, but we know that this took them time to develop. But more importantly, they had to spend time figuring out if this was even something worthwhile for them to do. Let's look at our communities first and review what our blood pressure numbers are. Can we find trends in our communities like they did? They had a clinic with patients in a nearby neighborhood all facing similar health issues. Based on our recent health status updates in our region, I know we have some possible opportunities. But, let's look into this further. And let's dig into our food challenges here. How many of our residents actually have access to the neighboring farmer's market? Is our issue a lack of farmer's markets, inconvenient hours, or is it that we could partner up with the neighboring city and do a better job of promoting what we already have in place? Is the real issue transportation? I think we have a lot of work to do before we jump into this idea." The volunteer nodded her head and said, "You know Sam. I get it. We really need to know what works here and what doesn't. Just because it would be a great idea to implement here doesn't mean it meets our needs. Maybe we need to develop our own version of this. I appreciate you and your insight. Thank you." Sam smiled and thanked the volunteers for sharing their ideas.

Activity 1.3: Discussion

After reviewing *Concept in Action 1.1,* how would you respond to each of the following questions?

1. What was your reaction to the volunteer approaching Sam with this idea? Should Sam have told the volunteer to wait until the next meeting to present it to everyone? Why or why not?
2. If you have not already reviewed the website, please do so and share your reaction to the program that was described.
3. What is your reaction to Sam's response? Why did Sam respond in this way?

struggling to pay their rent or mortgage, feed their family, or keep their family safe from the virus.

Current Challenges

Despite people living longer across the globe, there remain large gaps in health outcomes. Here are just a few of the types of health disparities that HES are needed to address and eliminate.

- WHO reports "a difference of 18 years of life expectancy between high- and low-income countries" and that the majority of the world's premature deaths as the result of noncommunicable or chronic diseases occur in low- and middle-income countries (2023b, Health Equity, para. 3).
- In the United States, deaths linked to heart disease, chronic lower respiratory disease, and stroke are higher in rural settings than in urban settings (National Heart Lung and Blood Institute [NHLBI], 2019).
- Colorectal cancer, lung cancer, and cervical cancer occur at higher rates in rural Appalachia when compared with neighboring urban settings (National Cancer Institute [NCI], 2022).
- Hispanic females born in 2015 have a life expectancy of 84.3 years, compared with 81.1 for non-Hispanic white females and 78.1 for non-Hispanic African American females (NHLBI, 2019).
- Cancer death rates are higher for Blacks and African Americans for most cancer types than any other race or ethnic group in the United States (NCI, 2022).
- Black and African Americans are more likely than white women to die from breast cancer (NCI, 2022).
- LGBTQ+ patients are more likely than non-LGBTQ+ patients to report "being blamed for health problems or having their concerns dismissed" (Dawson et al., 2021, para. 4).

These health disparities are complex and challenging. Yet, they do not capture all that makes individuals unique nor does it capture their full lived experiences. It is important to view health disparities and health equity with an understanding of intersectionality. **Intersectionality**, a term coined by Kimberlé Crenshaw, describes "how multiple identities interact to create unique patterns of oppression" (Gharib, 2022, para. 11). For example, consider the levels of discrimination that a Black Muslim woman who wears a hijab, lives below the poverty line, and uses a wheelchair may face. She will most likely face racism, religious discrimination, sexism, ableism, and source of income discrimination as she navigates through life. She will face obstacles and challenges in accessing services and obtaining the things she needs and wants in her life to succeed and thrive. These different forms of discrimination and the barriers that they create can significantly impact health outcomes.

In 2016, the National Collaborating Centre for Determinants of Health and the National Collaborating Centre for Healthy Public Policy, hosted a panel to explore ways that intersectionality is and can be applied to the practice of public health.

Samiya Abdi, a health promotion consultant who was part of a group interview, shared that "[t]his is an emerging field and public health needs to be at the forefront of it. We need to be brave enough to dream big and embrace the change or actually lead the change and see what policies can be put in place to support this in practice" (p. 8). To make this possible, it is necessary that HES are trained and prepared to do this work.

Today there are many HES in communities across the United States with the important job responsibility to deliver health education and promotion programs. However, not all of them are adequately prepared for their roles. Ensuring that HES are prepared to engage with individuals and communities in meaningful ways requires that they are equipped with essential skills to address current and emerging needs.

SIDEBAR: DID YOU KNOW?

Dr. Camara Jones, MD, MPH, PhD, is a family physician and epidemiologist who has dedicated her career to "naming, measuring, and addressing the impacts of racism on the health and well-being of the nation" (Emory University, 2022, para. 2) launched a national campaign against racism in 2016 while serving as the President of the American Public Health Association (APHA, 2023). Known for her love for storytelling, Dr. Jones uses allegories to explain racism.

Please visit https://www.youtube.com/watch?v=GNhcY6fTyBM to watch a 20-minute video where she shares four allegories to explain racism.

Activity 1.4: Practice Your Skills

Take a walk in your neighborhood, town, or campus and identify opportunities for health education and promotion. For example, some businesses will add signs by the elevator that encourage individuals to use the stairs instead. Perhaps you notice cigarette debris at the bus stop, which may be a potential opportunity to share smoking cessation information. See if you can find opportunities for health education and promotion for the four dimensions of health outlined in the chapter and then consider possible challenges with implementing any changes.

Summary

- The roles and responsibilities of a HES are varied. They range from developing and implementing health promotion programs to conducting research to advocacy. HES can be found in multiple settings with the overarching goal of promoting healthy behaviors that improve longevity and quality of life.

- Several key events occurred in the 20th century that helped to shape the health education and promotion profession. These include the Healthy People goals, the Ottawa Charter, and the CHES® and MCHES® certification.

- Health is more than the absence of an illness. The term *dimensions of health* is used to describe the various aspects of health. Most commonly, these dimensions include physical, spiritual, social, and psychological health. Optimal health is achieved when an individual has reached their highest level of wellness in any of the dimensions.

- Health disparities, differences in health outcomes, is a key focal point for HES throughout the United States. Communities now recognize that sustainable and effective improvements in health necessitate addressing and eliminating racism and other systemic barriers.

Web Resources
- **Healthy People 2030**
  https://health.gov/healthypeople
  Healthy People describes national objectives based on evidence-based recommendations to improve health outlined over a decade.
- **Racism and Health portal** (hosted by Centers for Disease Control and Prevention)
  https://www.cdc.gov/minorityhealth/racism-disparities/index.html
  This website provides links for readers to explore the specific research on the impact of racism on health outcomes, efforts by the CDC to address and ensure health equity, and provides information on why the CDC identified racism as a public health threat.
- **That's Public Health**
  https://www.apha.org/News-and-Media/Multimedia/Videos
  The American Public Health Association developed a video series that explores public health.
- **Unequal Treatment: Confronting Racial and Ethnic Disparities in Health Care**
  https://nap.nationalacademies.org/read/12875/chapter/1
  This landmark book demonstrates evidence of unequal treatment from healthcare professionals to people of color and how this leads to disparities in health outcomes. The PDF is free to download.

References

Abrams, E.M. & Szefler, S.J. (2020). COVID-19 and the impact of social determinants of health. *Lancet Respiratory Medicine*, 8(7), 659–661. https://doi.org/10.1016/S2213-2600(20)30234-4

American Medical Association. (2015). AMA Calls for Ban on DTC Ads of Prescription Drugs and Medical Devices. [Press Release]. https://www.ama-assn.org/press-center/press-releases/ama-calls-ban-dtc-ads-prescription-drugs-and-medical-devices

American Public Health Association. (2015). *The Role of Health Education Specialists in a Post-health Reform Environment* (Policy No. 201515). https://www.apha.org/policies-and-advocacy/public-health-policy-statements/policy-database/2016/01/27/13/58/role-of-health-education-specialists

American Public Health Association. (2021a). *Analysis: Declarations of Racism as a Public Health Crisis*. https://www.apha.org/-/media/Files/PDF/topics/racism/Racism_Declarations_Analysis.ashx

American Public Health Association. (2021b). *What Is Public Health?* https://www.apha.org/what-is-public-health

American Public Health Association. (2023). *Racial Equity*. https://www.apha.org/Topics-and-Issues/Racial-Equity

Blanding, M. (2022). *Revisiting the 'Unequal Treatment' Report, 20 Years Later*. https://harvardpublichealth.org/alumni-post/revisiting-the-unequal-treatment-report-20-years-later/

Buchmueller, T.C., Levinson, Z.M., Levy, H.G., & Wolfe, B.L. (2016). Effect of the Affordable Care Act on racial and ethnic disparities in health insurance coverage. *American Journal of Public Health*, 106(8), 1416–1421. https://doi.org/10.2105/AJPH.2016.303155

California Newsreel. (2008). *About the Series*. https://unnaturalcauses.org/about_the_series.php

Centers for Disease Control and Prevention. (2021a). Media Statement from CDC Director Rochelle P. Walensky, MD, MPH, on Racism and Health [Media Statement]. https://www.cdc.gov/media/releases/2021/s0408-racism-health.html

Centers for Disease Control and Prevention. (2021b). *Social Determinants of Health: Know What Affects Health.* https://www.cdc.gov/socialdeterminants/index.htm

Centers for Disease Control and Prevention. (2022). *About Chronic Diseases.* https://www.cdc.gov/socialdeterminants/index.htm

Centers for Disease Control and Prevention. (2023). *Physical Activity Helps Prevent Chronic Diseases.* https://www.cdc.gov/chronicdisease/index.htm#print

Commission on Social Determinants of Health. (2008). *Closing the Gap in a Generation: Health Equity through Action on the Social Determinants of Health.* Final Report of the Commission on Social Determinants of Health. Geneva, World Health Organization.

Dawson, L., Frederiksen, B., Long, M., Ranji, U. & Kates, J. (2021). LGBT+ People's Health and Experiences Accessing Care. KFF. https://www.kff.org/womens-health-policy/report/lgbt-peoples-health-and-experiences-accessing-care/

Emory University. (2022). *Camara Jones.* https://sph.emory.edu/faculty/profile/index.php?FID=camara-jones-8843

Gharib, S.E. (2022, Feb. 16). What is intersectionality and why is it important? *Global Citizen.* https://www.globalcitizen.org/en/content/what-is-intersectionality-explained/

History.com. (2009). *President Nixon Signs Legislation Banning Cigarette Ads on TV and Radio.* https://www.history.com/this-day-in-history/nixon-signs-legislation-banning-cigarette-ads-on-tv-and-radio

Huber, M. (2011). Health: How should we define it? *British Medical Journal, 343*(7817), 235–237. http://www.jstor.org/stable/23051314

Institute of Medicine. (2003). *Unequal Treatment: Confronting Racial and Ethnic Disparities in Health Care.* The National Academies Press. https://doi.org/10.17226/12875

Institute of Medicine (US) Committee on Educating Public Health Professionals for the 21st Century. (2003). History and current status of public health education in the United States. In K. Gebbie, L. Rosenstock, & L.M. Hernandez (Eds.), *Who Will Keep the Public Healthy? Educating Public Health Professionals for the 21st Century* (pp. 41–60). National Academies Press. https://www.ncbi.nlm.nih.gov/books/NBK221176/

Jadad, A.R. & O'Grady, L. (2008). What is health? The ability to adapt. *The Lancet, 373*(9666), 781. https://doi.org/10.1016/S0140-6736(09)60518-3

Merriam-Webster. (n.d.). Racism. In *Merriam-Webster.com dictionary.* Retrieved April 23, 2022, from https://www.merriam-webster.com/dictionary/racism

Milstein, S. & Karczmarczyk, D. (2021). Introduction to men's health. In D. Karczmarczyk & S. Milstein (Eds.), *Men's Health: An Introduction* (pp. 1–36). Routledge. https://doi.org/10.4324/9781351022620

National Association of Attorneys General. (2023). *The Master Settlement Agreement.* https://www.naag.org/our-work/naag-center-for-tobacco-and-public-health/the-master-settlement-agreement/

National Cancer Institute. (2022). *Cancer Disparities.* https://www.cancer.gov/about-cancer/understanding/disparities#:~:text=Black%2FAfrican%20American%20people%20have,to%20die%20of%20the%20disease

National Collaborating Centre for Determinants of Health & National Collaborating Centre for Healthy Public Policy. (2016). *Public Health Speaks: Intersectionality and Health Equity.* https://nccdh.ca/images/uploads/comments/Intersectionality_And_Health_Equity_EN_Mar24.pdf

National Commission for Health Education Credentialing, Inc. (n.d.-a). *List of Employers Who Hire/Recognize CHES® and MCHES®.* https://www.nchec.org/list-of-employers-who-hirerecognize-ches-and-mches

National Commission for Health Education Credentialing, Inc. (n.d.-b). *The Health Education Profession & Certification History Timeline.* https://www.nchec.org/profession

National Heart, Lung, and Blood Institute. (2019). *Health Disparities and Inequities.* https://www.nhlbi.nih.gov/science/health-disparities-and-inequities#:~:text=Differences%20in%20health%20among%20popu

National Library of Medicine. (n.d.). *The 1964 Report on Smoking and Health.* https://profiles.nlm.nih.gov/spotlight/nn/feature/smoking

Ochiai, E., Blakey, C., McGowan, A., & Lin, Y. (2021). The evolution of the healthy people initiative: A look through the decades. *Journal of Public Health Management and Practice, 27*(Suppl 6), S225–S234. https://doi.org/10.1097/PHH.0000000000001377

Office of Disease Prevention and Health Promotion. (n.d.-a). Health Equity in Healthy People 2030. *Healthy People 2030.* U.S. Department of Health and Human Services. https://health.gov/healthypeople/priority-areas/health-equity-healthy-people-2030

Office of Disease Prevention and Health Promotion. (n.d.-b). Social Determinants of Health. *Healthy People 2030.* U.S. Department of Health and Human Services, Office of Disease Prevention and Health Promotion. https://health.gov/healthypeople/objectives-and-data/social-determinants-health

Office of Minority Health. (n.d.). *National Culturally and Linguistically Appropriate Services Standards.* U.S. Department of Health and Human Services. https://thinkculturalhealth.hhs.gov/clas/standards

Prevention Research Center for Healthy Neighborhoods. (2020). *Produce Prescription Program (PRx).* http://prchn.org/prx/

Rimer, B.K., & Glanz, K. (2005). *Theory at a Glance: A Guide for Health Promotion Practice.* Bethesda, MD: US Department of Health and Human Services, National Institutes of Health, National Cancer Institute. https://www.sbccimplementationkits.org/demandrmnch/wp-content/uploads/2014/02/Theory-at-a-Glance-A-Guide-For-Health-Promotion-Practice.pdf?_ga=2.193644717.1427017897.1714334248-667860404.1714334248&_gl=1*8m52mf*_ga*NjY3ODYwNDA0LjE3MTQzMzQyNDg.*_ga_ETKXQ0SWKL*MTcxNDMzNDI0Ny4xLjAuMTcxNDMzNDI0Ny4wLjAuMA

Rooks, J.P. (2022). The history of midwifery. In Our Bodies Ourselves Today (Eds.), *Our Bodies Ourselves Today.* https://ourbodiesourselves.org/health-info/history-of-midwifery/

Rozen, A. (2022, March 5). *Q&A with Dr. Bill Hettler, MD, the Father of American Wellness.* https://www.linkedin.com/pulse/qa-dr-bill-hettler-md-father-american-wellness-adam-rozan

Social Security Online. (n.d.). *CES Report on Health Insurance: The Unpublished 1935 Report on Health Insurance & Disability.* Committee on Economic Security. http://www.socialsecurity.gov/history/reports/health.html

Temkin, O. (1940). Health education through the ages. *American Journal of Public Health, 30,* 1091–1095. https://www.ncbi.nlm.nih.gov/pmc/articles/PMC1531060/pdf/amjphnation00737-0077.pdf

Truth Initiative. (2017). *What do Tobacco Advertising Restrictions Look Like Today?* https://truthinitiative.org/research-resources/tobacco-industry-marketing/what-do-tobacco-advertising-restrictions-look-today

U.S. Bureau of Labor Statistics. (2022, April 22). *Occupational Outlook Handbook, Health Education Specialists and Community Health Workers.* https://www.bls.gov/ooh/community-and-social-service/health-educators.htm

U.S. Department of Health and Human Services. (2022). *About the Affordable Care Act.* https://www.hhs.gov/healthcare/about-the-aca/index.html

U.S. Office of the Surgeon General. (2023). *Our Epidemic of Loneliness and Isolation.* https://www.hhs.gov/sites/default/files/surgeon-general-social-connection-advisory.pdf

World Health Organization. (2009). *Milestones in Health Promotion: Statements from Global Conferences.* https://apps.who.int/iris/handle/10665/70578

World Health Organization. (2012). *Ottawa Charter for Health Promotion.* https://www.who.int/publications/i/item/WH-1987

World Health Organization. (2022). *Constitution.* https://www.who.int/about/governance/constitution

World Health Organization. (2023a). *About WHO.* https://www.who.int/about#:~:text=Founded%20in%201948%2C%20WHO%20is,the%20highest%20level%20of%20health

World Health Organizations. (2023b). *Social Determinants of Health.* https://www.who.int/health-topics/social-determinants-of-health#tab=tab_1

Yale University Library. (2003). *Selling Smoke: Tobacco Advertising and Anti-smoking Campaigns.* https://onlineexhibits.library.yale.edu/s/sellingsmoke/page/science/

CHAPTER 2

Essential Skills and Competencies: Setting Strong Foundations

Learning Objectives

After reading this chapter, learners will be able to:

- **Compare the eight Areas of Responsibility developed by the National Commission for Health Education Credentialing for HES job functions**
- **Describe the skills necessary for successful programming efforts in population health and systems-based approaches**
- **Explain the requirements and process of obtaining a CHES® or MCHES® credential**

Keywords

- Areas of Responsibility
- Certified Health Education Specialist – CHES®
- Code of Ethics for the Health Education Profession®
- Competencies
- Master Certified Health Education Specialist – MCHES®
- National Commission for Health Education Credentialing, Inc.
- Sub-competencies

Self-Reflection Questions

Take a moment and reflect on these questions:
1. What skills do HES need to be effective in their role?
2. What are the benefits for seeking a certification as a CHES® or MCHES®?

DOI: 10.4324/9781003504320-2

There are many job and career opportunities in public health. Each of these requires a set of skills and subject matter expertise to be effective. The **National Commission for Health Education Credentialing, Inc.** (NCHEC) has identified specific skills needed to be successful as a HES. These skills are organized into eight **Areas of Responsibility** with specific **competencies** and **sub-competencies**. These competencies and sub-competencies are assessed through a national certification process that can result in becoming credentialed HES.

This chapter will review these eight Areas, provide examples of related skills, and explain how these skills are utilized every day by HES. In addition, this chapter will explore the process for becoming a Certified Health Education Specialist (CHES®) and a master-level CHES®, referred to as MCHES®. Finally, this chapter will explore how the practice of ethical behavior encompasses all competencies to ensure health education and promotion professionals are sufficiently prepared for their roles.

Role of NCHEC

NCHEC was incorporated in 1988 to "address the industry-wide need to enhance the professional practice of Health Education through the promotion of a credentialed body of Health Education Specialists" (National Commission for Health Education Credentialing [NCHEC], n.d.-a, para. 3). In addition, NCHEC administers the CHES® and MCHES® exams which are based on a comprehensive analysis – referred to as a "practice analysis study" (para. 1) (NCHEC, n.d.-e). This analysis is conducted every five years through a national survey of health education and promotion professionals from a variety of worksites and sectors to determine the current and accurate skills utilized by and necessary for health education professionals in the workplace (NCHEC, n.d.-a, n.d.-e). A task force analyzes the results and updates a "framework for the profession" that can be used by HES as well as academics who work to ensure both undergraduate- and graduate-level programs in health education and promotion are including these skills in their respective programs (NCHEC, n.d.-e, para. 2). The framework is also used to develop the exam to certify entry-level skills through the CHES® exam and those that are considered to be more advanced through the MCHES® exam (NCHEC, n.d.-e).

Eight Areas of Responsibility

The most recent analysis, the Health Education Specialist Practice Analysis II, was completed in 2020 (NCHEC, n.d.-f). As a result of this most recent analysis, the seven Areas of Responsibility were revised to **Eight Areas of Responsibility** with competencies and sub-competencies for each (NCHEC, 2019). In addition, Advocacy and Communication were included as separate Areas, and emphasis was placed on the increasing importance of social media in public health in the development of the competencies and sub-competencies (NCHEC, 2019).

The eight Areas of Responsibility (as indicated in Table 2.1) include Area I: Assessment of Needs and Capacity, Area II: Planning, Area III: Implementation, Area IV: Evaluation and Research, Area V: Advocacy, Area VI: Communication, Area VII: Leadership and Management, and Area VIII: Ethics and Professionalism (NCHEC, n.d.-e). Within

Table 2.1 Eight Areas of Responsibility for CHES® and MCHES®

Areas of Responsibility	
Area I: Assessment of needs and capacity	Area V: Advocacy
Area II: Planning	Area VI: Communication
Area III: Implementation	Area VII: Leadership and management
Area IV: Evaluation and research	Area VIII: Ethics and professionalism

Note: Adapted from "Responsibilities and Competencies for Health Education Specialists" by National Commission for Health and Education Credentialing, Inc., n.d.-e, para. 4. Retrieved from https://www.nchec.org/responsibilities-and-competencies

each Area, NCHEC describes in detail each Area by listing related Competencies (35) and Sub-competencies (193). Competencies are the main job functions that entry-level HES are expected to be able to perform on the job. Sub-competencies are more detailed job expectations within each Competency. To differentiate between different levels of experience and practice, some Sub-competencies are categorized as advanced (NCHEC, 2020).

Although the NCHEC's eight Areas of Responsibility provide a general list of competencies and sub-competencies for HES, examples of how these competencies and sub-competencies are represented on the job are not included. In the next section, each Area will be introduced with examples of the job duties HES may have as part of their professional role.

> **SIDEBAR: DID YOU KNOW?**
>
> The number of competencies and sub-competencies for each Area of Responsibility varies. To review the eight Areas and each of the related competencies and sub-competencies, please visit: https://www.nchec.org/responsibilities-and-competencies.

Area I: Assessment of Needs and Capacity

Each of the Areas identified by NCHEC is important. Area I is important because knowing the needs of a community before health education and promotion interventions or programs begin is essential to ensuring that they address the actual needs of the community. HES will need to consider:

- What data is available to determine the current health status of the community?
- Is the data readily available or does data need to be collected?
- What interventions, programs, or services are needed to improve the health of the community?

Once data is identified and collected, HES and other invested partners must analyze and interpret the data. In this later step, capacity can be gauged to determine if the community has the personnel, dedicated time and resources, and overall infrastructure to support needed change.

Assessing Communities

The topic of assessing communities and the skills required to do this effectively is explored in Chapter 3. The topic will include examples of how HES assess communities and how this information is used to improve health outcomes.

This Area includes job activities such as starting a local health coalition on physical activity composed of groups of people who collaborate to work on this issue or problem. HES may conduct key informant interviews about the transportation needs of older adults. The information obtained in these interviews can be used to improve access to needed programs and services. HES may look at very specific data, such as tobacco use, and then write a report to compare their findings to local, regional, and national tobacco use data. This report might be used to secure funding, provide rationale for more resources, or document health disparities for baseline measurements. Overall, a needs assessment process guides the work of HES and communities in advancing health outcomes strategically and logically.

Area II: Planning

Planning is another key role for HES. Health education and promotion interventions, programs, and services must be intentionally designed to meet the identified needs and gaps of a population. To be most successful, planning efforts are a collaborative process that involves community partners and other invested groups. When combined with a robust needs assessment process, planning ensures that the interventions chosen will lead to the best health outcomes.

Planning Interventions and Programs

The topic of planning interventions and programs is explored in Chapter 5. This chapter includes an exploration of the many resources available to HES to do this effectively.

This Area includes job activities such as developing goals and objectives. This is important because there needs to be a purpose for each intervention, program, or service. The purpose needs to be reflected in an overall goal and the objectives are the action steps to meeting the goal. For example, by the end of a four-week tobacco prevention program, how many students are you hoping will have completed the educational modules? Another job activity for HES in this Area includes drafting language to justify grant funding for a proposed intervention or program. HES might be tasked with writing the rationale section of a grant application. After securing funding, HES could also be tasked with researching and developing the proposed project. For example, if the grant proposal that was awarded included the development of an after-school program on gardening for elementary school children, then HES may be responsible for making that happen.

Area III: Implementation

Once planning is complete and interventions chosen, program implementation can begin. This is the skill captured in Area III. HES could be directly involved with implementation or have a more coordinating and monitoring role. This means utilizing skills in project management. An example of coordinating may also be when the implementation of a program requires formal training for the program leaders. This may happen when the program that is being implemented is an existing program that is being replicated, with permission or purchase of a curriculum. Sometimes, curricula may need to be developed and HES may be responsible for supporting those who are developing it or may be drafting content themselves. Overall, HES are often responsible for the key details of the successful implementation of health education and promotion programs.

Implementing Interventions and Programs

The topic of implementing interventions and programs is also explored in Chapter 5.

In preparation for implementing a health intervention or program, HES job activities may include ordering and purchasing necessary supplies. For example, a nutrition education program that includes a cooking demonstration needs supplies such as the ingredients, paper products to offer samples to those attending, and cookware. HES could also teach an eight-session program on falls prevention to older adults, including ways to make their home safer and strength and balance exercises they can do at home. This means that they would need to take attendance, teach each session, and be available for follow-up questions from participants. Because HES often work in teams, they may assist another HES or colleague in conducting an HIV testing event at a local university by conducting intake sessions or offering mini-educational sessions on safe sex practices. Implementing programs includes the delivery and execution of interventions and programs. Being organized, having the necessary supplies and training materials, or monitoring the level of engagement by participants are all aspects of this Area.

Area IV: Evaluation and Research

Area IV is about evaluation and research. In order to demonstrate and prove that a health education and health promotion program was a success, it must be evaluated. Evaluations can also identify challenges and barriers in implementation. Effective and useful evaluations consist of a well-designed research plan to analyze process, impact, and outcome measures through the collection of data. HES must be able to appropriately design the research study that will yield the data that is needed to evaluate the program. Once data is collected, it must be interpreted and then presented in a useful format. For example, this type of information is often needed to produce reports and other documents for members of the community, funders, elected officials, and others who are interested in seeing the results and impact of specific interventions, programs, and services.

Evaluating Interventions and Programs

The topic of evaluation is explored in Chapter 4. The reason that this is covered before planning and implementation is because developing an evaluation of interventions and programs
needs to occur as part of the planning process to be included as part of successful implementation efforts.

One job activity that HES might be responsible for in this Area includes creating a
pre- and post-survey to be used as part of the evaluation of a curriculum on prevention of bullying in high schools. HES may be asked to disseminate the surveys, collect
them, analyze the results, and draft a written report for the funder or School Board.
HES often collaborate with others as part of their role. When tasked with drafting the
evaluation section in a grant proposal, HES could reach out to a local university for
assistance with identifying an evaluation plan. Faculty and students at colleges and
universities are often interested in partnering on projects that provide them with the
opportunity to be more involved in the community. Another example of a job activity in this Area is presenting the results of a community-wide program on decreasing
pedestrian deaths to the City Council as they consider legislation and budget alloca-
tions on crosswalks and speed zones. Additional presentations might be requested by
law enforcement, bicycle advocates, and parents. These examples demonstrate that this
Area includes identifying an evaluation plan, conducting the evaluation, and using the
results of the evaluation to inform others.

Area V: Advocacy

HES are often deeply committed and invested in the community that they are serving
and are frequently called upon to be an advocate. For example, a needs assessment may
have revealed health issues that need urgent attention and need more resources directed
to them. HES may work with community organizers and others to educate those in
decision-making roles on funding and policies and how different strategies for addressing the issues can be helpful. Successful advocacy includes reaching out to stakeholders;
providing current, accurate, and timely education; and following up with an evaluation
of how effective the advocacy efforts were.

Advocacy

The topic of advocacy is explored in Chapter 6.

Because HES are often considered subject matter experts in a variety of community health issues, HES might write talking points for coalition members to use when
meeting with elected officials. HES might take the lead on coordinating meetings with
elected officials about a dangerous intersection in the community that needs a traffic

signal and an updated crosswalk. Parents and school administrators could be interested partners in these types of initiatives. Making these connections and establishing relationships are key parts of advocacy. Another example of a job activity is for HES to write a report that documents the advocacy efforts of a local task force on water run-off from a manufacturing plant to solicit financial support from a funder. The report could also include data on water quality and be presented at a neighborhood meeting.

Area VI: Communication

Area VI is about communication. This includes developing and disseminating messages designed to improve health and keep individuals and communities safe. For example, during the early days and months of the COVID-19 pandemic, lots of messages about health risks were circulating. Some of this information was misleading and inaccurate and some was accurate and helpful. Providing clear, concise, and actionable health messages can be the difference between life and death. Before messages can be developed and tested, HES need to know how their target audiences best receive health communication. For some, it might be social media. For others, the best medium might be text messages or even a door-to-door campaign. Regardless of the channel used, like all other components of a health intervention, communication activities need to be evaluated.

Communication

The topic of communication is explored in Chapter 7.

There are many examples of communication job activities that are conducted by HES. For example, HES may conduct a focus group on three public service announcements created to increase breastfeeding in a low-income area to test if the message resonates with community members and is clear. HES need to utilize their knowledge on the Social Determinants of Health to inform their work. Does it make sense to have a message on breastfeeding only at bus stops or would it be more effective if local businesses helped to promote the message? Should the message be offered in multiple languages? HES could be interviewed by the local television station on the seasonal flu shot campaign. The campaign might include using messaging from state and national partners, such as the Centers for Disease Control and Prevention. HES need to identify the most important message for the medium and the time allotted. So, a 3-minute interview needs to be very specific to be effective. Another communication example is to research, develop, and create social media posts for a short-term campaign on drinking and driving during prom and graduation season. HES may also be responsible for posting the messages and interacting with those who respond. The Area of communication is one that requires the ability to create and distribute messages proactively on health topics and react when appropriate. For example, HES may post messages about a community incident and provide resources in mental health services in that area to be responsive to the immediate need for support. HES may also develop messages based on monthly themes, such as popular awareness month themes like diabetes and heart health. Finally, HES may create content that is longer such as a video script or podcast on a health topic. There are many types of job activities for HES in this Area.

Area VII: Leadership and Management

As HES advance in their professional skills and responsibilities, they may assume management and leadership roles within their organization. Developing and maintaining professional relationships are important components of effective management and aid in the success of an effective leader. Relationships with key community partners are invaluable and much needed to accomplish the work of a HES. Relationships take time to develop and nurture. These relationships need to be authentic and genuine. Leaders will also be called upon to mentor others in health education and promotion, and share their experience and expertise. In addition to managing people, leaders need to be able to oversee and direct financial and material resources. Finally, HES will be invited to participate in, if not lead, strategic planning processes. These may be internal to an organization, such as a health department, or external for a hospital system or community, and they may be for short-term goals or long-term plans. For example, HES may have to develop a five-year strategic plan for their unit.

> **Leadership**
>
> The topic of leadership is explored in Chapter 5.

As leaders in public health, HES might serve on an expert panel on the community's health at a town hall meeting. HES may be invited to serve in a leadership role at regional Task Force to address gun violence or serve as a member of Board to advise on physical activity for youth. Sitting on a strategic planning committee for the local hospital is another example of a HES in a leadership role within the community. As a manager, HES can identify staffing needs for their department, draft job descriptions, identify and interview, hire, and train entry and mid-level health education and promotion professionals for a new grant-funded program on school-based nutrition. This will also require identifying the qualifications needed for this role.

Area VIII: Ethics and Professionalism

Of the eight Areas, Area VIII is the newest and focuses on ethics and professionalism (NCHEC, 2019). Merriam-Webster defines ethics as, "the principles of conduct governing an individual or a group" (2023, para. 2). Ethics describes behavior as morally right – truthful, fair, and honest. Performing one's work duties in an ethical manner is paramount to the work that HES do on a daily basis. Without trust, HES are unable to represent themselves as true agents of change. While frequently serving as a resource for health information, HES are responsible for people's health and many times, their quality of life. It is a big responsibility and not one to be taken lightly. HES also need to pay attention to changes and new developments in public health and science. Continuing education and professional development activities are designed to keep HES on the cutting edge of what works and what does not.

Ethics

The topic of ethics is explored in multiple chapters, including Chapters 2 and 8.

One example where fairness and justice might play a role is if a HES has to make a decision on which school will receive a small grant to upgrade their athletic fields. In some instances, schools with higher family income levels may already have advantages over other schools. Making the decision on which school receives the grant may seem like a simple decision to make; however, there may be hidden implications of the decision. For example, will this small grant make the school ineligible to receive funding from other sources that may actually be higher in amount? HES will need to explore ways to make the best-informed decision, ideally with the input of interested parties. Another way HES might explore just actions is to help inform the community at large about health equity issues and write a blog post or be interviewed for a podcast. Finally, this Area also includes the expectations of a health education and promotion professional to disseminate their findings to the broader public health field and share their subject matter expertise. This might include presenting the results of a program on youth obesity at a national public health conference or collaborating with a state-wide coalition as an expert on health promotion strategies related to preventing tobacco use among youth.

A Focus on Ethics

The Coalition for National Health Education Organizations (CNHEO) maintains and regularly updates the **Code of Ethics for the Health Education Profession**® (Code) for the health education and promotion profession (2020).

Eight Areas of Responsibility for CHES® and MCHES®

Acting as an ethical professional aligns with the following Areas of Responsibility for CHES® and MCHES®:

Area VIII: Ethics and Professionalism

This area includes four competencies and 21 sub-competencies detailing the expectations of CHES® and MCHES® throughout their career (National Commission for Health and Education Credentialing, Inc. [NCHEC], 2020). This includes knowing existing ethical guidelines and using them appropriately in the profession, being available as a health education and health promotion resource, participating in ongoing professional development to stay up to date with current research and best practices, and advocating for the field of health education and promotion (NCHEC, 2020).

To learn more about the Areas of Responsibility, please visit https://www.nchec.org/.

The Code emphasizes a shared framework of guiding concepts, such as valuing life, justice, beneficence, and the avoidance of harm. HES have a responsibility to maintain high levels of professional behavior for themselves as well as their colleagues, clients, and stakeholders. The primary role of HES is to promote health in a variety of settings, from individuals to communities to organizations. By believing in and following the Code, HES can ensure that they are working to ensure that their work values and appreciates all of the different people with whom they interact. The Code is to be used when making work-related decisions.

Activity 2.1: Discussion

Review the Code of Ethics for the Health Education Profession® and consider the following scenarios. What ethical dilemma(s) can you identify?

Link to the Code: https://drive.google.com/file/d/1tMIqPXW3ruG9FQoAXHkf6VdEKqGibEmP/view

1. Suppose that you are a HES leading an education seminar with a fellow HES. At the end of the session, you welcome questions from the audience. A community member shares a detailed description of symptoms that they have been experiencing for the past few months. Your colleague interrupts the community members and says, "Based on what you just shared with me, I know that you definitely have a traumatic brain injury and it's getting worse. I have no doubt about it. Let's talk about what medical steps you need to take as someone with that kind of injury after we end the session."
2. You decided to swap resumes with a fellow HES as you are both looking for feedback as you begin a job search. You notice that your colleague has claimed that they have earned a specific certification and have it listed on their resume. When you ask them about it they share, "Oh! Yeah, I don't actually have that certification but I know that it will look better on my resume if I list it."
3. Your boss has asked you to work on recruiting program participants for a grant-funded project. Because of time constraints, you are told to not worry about obtaining informed consent and that you can do that at the end of the program.

CHES® and MCHES® Exams

The CHES® and MCHES® exams are administered by NCHEC. The first certification exam to credential Certified Health Education Specialists occurred in 1990 with the CHES® exam (NCHEC, n.d.-f). The CHES® exam was initially offered once a year, moving to twice a year in 1997, and now offered for a period of a few days during two months of the year (NCHEC, n.d.-f). In 2011, the Master Certified Health Education Specialist (MCHES®) exam was offered (NCHEC, n.d.-f) for professionals seeking an advanced-level certification. Both the CHES® and MCHES® exams are "the ONLY nationally and

> **SIDEBAR: DID YOU KNOW?**
>
> For the most recent and up-to-date information on the CHES® and MCHES® exams, the NCHEC website is the best resource. Please visit: https://www.nchec.org/

internationally accredited certifications in the public/community health education arena" (NCHEC, n.d.-a, para. 25). According to NCHEC, "[the] CHES® and MCHES® certifications create a national and international standard for health education specialists practicing at both entry and advanced levels" (NCHEC, n.d.-d, para. 1).

Eligibility Requirements

Eligibility requirements for the CHES® exam include a bachelor's degree or higher in Health Education, or a related degree plus 25 credits specifically in Health Education (NCHEC, n.d.-b). The CHES® credential is specific to health education and promotion and is specifically designed for individuals in the early stages of their profession (NCHEC, n.d.-a). This credential is appropriate for those who assist with community needs assessments and developing community health improvement plans, select participants and deliver training, and help to collect and analyze data for program evaluation and similar tasks (NCHEC, n.d.-a).

Eligibility requirements for the MCHES® exam include a master's degree and at least five years of health education and promotion experience (NCHEC, n.d.-b). A candidate for the MCHES® exam may also qualify for this advanced-level certification by holding the CHES® credential for at least five years (NCHEC, n.d.-b). This advanced credential is designed for experienced HES who, as part of their daily job functions, hire and train other HES, design and develop program budgets, apply ethical principles to real-world situations, and develop and monitor strategic plans (NCHEC, n.d.-a). The differences between the two credentials are summarized in Table 2.2.

Test Format

These exams are based on the eight Areas of Responsibility. As a result of the recent analysis, as of April 2023, the exams moved from questions covering the seven Areas of Responsibility to covering the eight Areas of Responsibility with the corresponding

Table 2.2 Comparison of CHES® and MCHES® Examination by Audience, Content, and Job Duties

Exam	Audience	Content	Job Duties
CHES® Exam	Early career professional	Entry-level competencies	Select training participants, deliver training, and identify potential program evaluation tools
MCHES® Exam	Advanced career professional with at least five years of experience	Advanced-level competencies and sub-competencies	Develop and manage budgets, apply ethical principles, identify staff development and training needs, and develop and monitor strategic plan

Note: Adapted from "Overview" by NCHEC, n.d.-c, para. 2 and para. 3. Retrieved from https://www.nchec.org/overview

Competencies and Sub-competencies for each (NCHEC, n.d.-b). The CHES® examination contains 165 multiple-choice questions; 150 are scored and 15 are not scored (NCHEC, n.d.-d). The questions that are not scored are questions that are being considered for future exams. The exam must be completed within three hours (NCHEC, n.d.-d). Both exams are only offered in a computer-based format to be completed at professional test centers or at home with prior approval (NCHEC, n.d.-d). Candidates can choose which test center is best for them when applying for the exam. In 2022, 68.5% of candidates who took the CHES® exam passed and 62.7% of candidates who took the MCHES® exam passed (NCHEC, n.d.-d).

NCHEC continues to show solid growth in certifying both CHES® and MCHES®. The 2022 exam cycle had a total of 2,261 CHES® registrants and 199 MCHES® registrants (n.d.-d). Overall, NCHEC reports that combined there are over 15,100 CHES® and MCHES® "representing all 50 states in the United States, Puerto Rico, as well as many others who are practicing internationally or on military bases overseas" (n.d.-d, para. 8).

Concept in Action 2.1

Background: *Tasha* (she/her) is an entry-level HES with a Bachelor's degree in Community Health. She is employed at the local hospital. Tasha's supervisor told her that the hospital would pay for her to take the CHES® exam because it is now a requirement for her position. Tasha remembers hearing about the CHES® exam in college but she did not think she needed to take it right after she graduated. She has now been on the job for about a year and is interested in taking the exam to demonstrate that she has the knowledge and skill set to succeed. She wonders if her work responsibilities to date have prepared her to take the exam.

Tasha has many questions at this stage. These include:

1. Do I have the qualifications to take the exam?
2. How can I best prepare for the exam? What should I study?
3. When, where, and how do I register and take the exam?
4. What happens if I do not pass the exam?

To help her prepare for the exam, Tasha purchased the study guide from the NCHEC website and joined a study group with some of her peers from college who will also be taking the exam.

Job Requirements

Employers in the United States may indicate a preference or requirement for hiring HES with a CHES® or MCHES® certification in position descriptions (NCHEC, n.d.-c). Typically, this is indicated either in the qualifications section (as indicated in Figure 2.1) or at the end of the advertisement. Sometimes employers will specify that the candidate must obtain the CHES® or MCHES® certification within a specified time after they are hired. Having a CHES® or MCHES® certification at the time of hire may be an advantage in a hiring process and is strongly recommended to those who plan on working in the health education and promotion field.

Health Promotion Specialist

Job Number: BBT-0988

Location: Anytown, USA

Workplace-type: Hybrid, work from home 3 days per week

*Note: This position requires travel within assigned area 60% of the time for meetings and conferences

The Company has an excellent opportunity for a **Health Promotion Specialist.** Working as a member of the Health Promotions & Education department, you will join an outstanding group of professionals dedicated to our mission: to save lives by improving community health and preventing chronic disease through research, education, and advocacy. In this role you will oversee and coordinate youth-led movements. **This position is grant-funded for 3 years**

Responsibilities:

- Recruit, establish, and provide direction for youth involved in the project
- Establish work plans for projects that address the needs of youth
- Manage the project website and social media channels
- Host training sessions for youth groups on advocacy
- Develop technical assistance resources to help project advisors successfully implement youth programming
- Compile information about project numbers and activities for the year for the annual report
- Compile information about project numbers and activities for the quarterly report
- Compile and distribute the Biannual Advisor Survey
- Participate in monthly project calls to discuss youth program updates and share ideas
- Participate in monthly check in calls with the project funder
- Create/distribute the monthly and quarterly e-newsletter via Constant Contact
- Schedule and hold regular volunteer meetings
- Conduct evaluation activities and reporting across youth programs, ensuring timely and accurate submission of individual-level data reporting as required by the Company and funding sources
- Present program outcomes and disseminate surveillance and evaluation findings at statewide and national meetings, as needed
- Represent the Company as a member of community, civic, and/or health coalitions and organizations related to the Company's mission
- Build, maintain, and cultivate relationships with funders, facilitators, community partners, other youth coalitions, and national partners to encourage program delivery, sustainability, and growth across service territory
- Select and participate in local, state, and national seminars and courses designed to increase skills and knowledge related to job requirements
- Participate in and support all area events and provide support for annual reports, awards, grants and other activities as assigned

Qualifications:

- Bachelor's Degree in public health, health education, health promotion, or related field or equivalent combination of education and work experience required
- CHES® and/or MCHES® is preferred
- Minimum two years of experience developing and implementing community awareness, education, stakeholder engagement, and programs specifically related to areas of public health
- Prior experience in public health, social services, public policy, and/or advocacy required
- Must be a self-starter with excellent communication skills both written and oral
- Positive attitude with the ability to work independently and cooperatively in a team environment
- Must have a valid Driver's license and reliable transportation to travel within assigned area 60% of the time for meetings and conferences, and flexibility to work irregular hours, including evenings and weekends with some overnights required
- Able to work with minimum direct supervision, make decisions, and take initiative
- Proven ability to cultivate and steward relationships across a diverse population
- Must be proficient in Microsoft Office and internet applications
- Ability to lift up to 25 pounds
- Consistent with its mission, the Company maintains a smoke-free workplace, all employees must abstain from using tobacco in any form, including vaping

Application Procedure:

To apply, email a cover letter, resume, and salary requirements (include the job title and the job number in the subject of the email) to humanresources@company.org.

The Company is dedicated to a diverse workforce.
Equal Opportunity Employer EOE/M/F/D/V/SO

Benefits: The Company offers a comprehensive benefits package that includes: Medical, Dental, Vision, Employee Assistance Program, Paid Parental Leave FSA, HSA, LTD, STD, Life insurance, AD&D, Matching 401(k), Paid Vacation/Sick/Holidays.

Salary: The target hiring range for this position is between $46,000 and $51,000.

Figure 2.1 Sample job description.

Activity 2.2: Discussion

Review the job description in Figure 2.1 and discuss the following questions:

1. Does the job title appeal to you? Why or why not?
2. What are the implications of a grant-funded position?
3. What are the main job duties listed? Does this job seem realistic to you?
4. What are the education requirements? Is there a certification required?
5. Do you feel qualified to apply to this job description? If not, why?
6. What do you need to help prepare you for this position?
7. What are your thoughts on the benefits and salary range?

Summary

■ There are essential skills and competencies for professionals working in health education and promotion, this includes professionals working in community health, global health, and wellness. The roles and responsibilities of HES are varied. NCHEC published the eight Areas of Responsibility to outline these roles and provide detailed Competencies and Sub-competencies necessary to perform the functions of HES. The Areas, competencies, and competencies are reviewed and updated every five years and serve as the cogent basis for the CHES® and MCHES® exams.

■ The skills HES utilize are varied. They range from developing and implementing health promotion programs to conducting research to advocacy. HES can be found in multiple settings with the overarching goal of promoting healthy behaviors that improve longevity and quality of life.

■ The CHES® and MCHES® credentials are designed to provide HES with proof of their knowledge and skills. Specific academic preparation in health education and promotion or prior CHES® credentials is required to be eligible for each exam. HES who pass the exams can be proud of their accomplishments and use their credentials to set them apart from other job candidates.

Web Resources

■ **National Commission for Health Education Credentialing, Inc. (NCHEC)**
https://www.nchec.org
The CHES® and MCHES® examinations and certifications are administered by NCHEC.

■ **O*Net OnLine: Health Education Specialists**
https://www.onetonline.org/link/summary/21-1091.00
The U.S. Department of Labor, Employment and Training Administration provides updated information about various occupations, including required skills, education, and the projected job outlook.

References

Coalition for National Health Education Organizations. (2020). *Code of Ethics for the Health Education Profession®*. https://www.cnheo.org/files/coe_full_2011.pdf

Merriam-Webster. (2023). Ethic. In *Merriam-Webster.com dictionary*. Retrieved August 19, 2023, from https://www.merriam-webster.com/dictionary/ethic

National Commission for Health and Education Credentialing, Inc. (n.d.-a). *CHES®/MCHES®*. https://www.nchec.org/cph-and-ches?source=adwords&campaign=&medium=cpc&keyword=&target=dsa-19959388920&loc=9008183&device=c&gclid=Cj0KCQjwkruVBh-CHARIsACVIiOzwanJDMAFftF33mlZdZZt3x_l-MNzCQ1RcjxsFNEagH-3KQGyeqNIaAhGmEALw_wcB

National Commission for Health and Education Credentialing, Inc. (n.d.-b). *CHES Exam*. https://www.nchec.org/ches-exam-eligibility

National Commission for Health Education Credentialing, Inc. (n.d.-c). *List of Employers Who Hire/Recognize CHES® and MCHES®*. https://www.nchec.org/list-of-employers-who-hirerecognize-ches-and-mches

National Commission for Health and Education Credentialing, Inc. (n.d.-d). *Overview*. https://www.nchec.org/overview

National Commission for Health and Education Credentialing, Inc. (n.d.-e). *Responsibilities and Competencies for Health Education Specialists*. https://www.nchec.org/responsibilities-and-competencies

National Commission for Health and Education Credentialing, Inc. (n.d.-f). *The Health Education Profession & Certification History Timeline*. https://www.nchec.org/profession

National Commission for Health and Education Credentialing, Inc. (2019, September 30). *Health Education Specialist Practice Analysis II 2020 Validates and reveals Eight Areas of Responsibility for Health Education Specialists* [Press release]. https://assets.speakcdn.com/assets/2251/hespa_ii_press_release_-_web_final_0520.pdf

National Commission for Health and Education Credentialing, Inc. (2020). *Areas of Responsibility, Competencies and Sub-competencies for Health Education Specialist Practice Analysis II 2020 (HESPA II 2020)*. https://assets.speakcdn.com/assets/2251/hespa_competencies_and_sub-competencies_052020.pdf

CHAPTER 3

Assessing Communities: Understanding the Needs and Gaps

Keywords

- Community
- Community Health Assessment aNd Group Evaluation (CHANGE)
- Community Health Improvement Plan
- Community Health Needs Assessment
- Comorbidities
- Enabling Factors
- Evidence-Based Interventions
- Health Needs
- Health Outcomes

- Intervention
- Mobilizing for Action through Planning and Partnerships model (MAPP)
- Morbidity
- PRECEDE-PROCEED Model
- Predisposing Factors
- Qualitative Data
- Quantitative Data
- Reinforcing Factors
- Windshield Tour

DOI: 10.4324/9781003504320-3

> **Self-Reflection Questions**
> Take a moment and reflect on these questions:
> 1. What is one community you are a part of?
> 2. What do you think are the top three health needs in your community?
> 3. Would everyone else in your community agree that these are the top three health needs? Why or why not?

A **community** can be defined as any group of individuals who share a common purpose, location, or situation. Individuals can be a part of multiple communities. The term community can also be used to collectively recognize the diversity in the various types of community spaces that HES may work in. This can include, but not be limited to, a college campus, a specific town or city, or a company. Each of these communities has its own identities, resources, and needs.

An important role of a HES is to improve health outcomes, regardless of the community. **Health outcomes** are the improvements seen in health. Depending on the issue, this can be either an increase or a decrease. For example, an improved health outcome in terms of smoking would be a *decrease* in the number of adolescents who initiate smoking. An improved health outcome can also be an increase, such as an *increase* in the number of vegetables adults report consuming during the week. There are many health outcomes that could be identified and addressed in any community. While some health outcomes require years to achieve, sometimes there is an immediate health need that requires attention. For example, if HES are employed by a local school and the school experiences an outbreak of norovirus, a contagious virus that can cause diarrhea, HES may create a program promoting hand washing to help curb future infections. In this case, the need is clear and requires a rapid response. In this example, there is a communicable disease that is impacting the school. However, the health needs of a community may not often be as clear or as simple to address. Health concerns in a community can also include a high rate of obesity, smoking, and the incidence of colorectal cancer. It could include the lack of available mental health resources and the rising rates of suicides. These health concerns, also referred to as **health needs**, are a bit more complex. This chapter will review how to determine health needs in a community using various models and strategies, and how to prioritize the health needs to decide on the next steps. Finally, the chapter will provide limitations of needs assessments and how these limitations impact population health outcomes.

Exploring Health Needs

Let's consider the topic of smoking. Why do individuals smoke or use tobacco products? There can be many reasons, including addiction to nicotine. A common reason individuals indicate that they use tobacco products is to help with stress management. Therefore, a more meaningful approach to address smoking, or tobacco use, may be to address effective stress management. Identifying why an individual is engaging in a particular health behavior can help to identify a root cause. A **root cause** is best described as the explanation for why the behavior started in the first place. For example, what are the sources of stress? Are the stressors cumulative or temporary? These all may help to explain what might be helpful to aid in cessation. Being intentional and meaningful in health promotion efforts is an important part of developing tailored interventions. An **intervention** is a program, policy, or service that is created or maintained to address health behaviors and improve health outcomes. The term intervention is often used interchangeably with health promotion programs.

Terminology in This Book

The term intervention is used in this book to refer to a health promotion project, program, service, or policy.

HES are prepared to dig into health needs to try and understand the associated behaviors to ensure that the interventions that are developed can be successful. For example, tobacco use may occur among friends or multiple members of a family. This may make quitting even more difficult as there may be other individuals whose smoking behavior may make it challenging to quit alone. So, an intervention aimed at quitting should include addressing peer and family influences.

Developing Interventions

Planning and implementing interventions are further explored in Chapter 5.

Community Health Needs Assessments

Interventions should be designed to address health needs within a community. They may address one specific topic or a myriad of health needs. In reality, there are many possible health needs within a community. To gain an understanding of what these are, it is important to identify what the current health status is of a community and where opportunity exists for improvement. A **Community Health Needs Assessment**, often referred to as a Community Health Assessment (CHA), is a systematic process for doing just that. This process uses various strategies to identify and collect data to understand the community, its health status, and top health needs. This process also includes identifying the priority topics to be addressed. This does not mean that health needs that are not identified are ignored, it is just that they are not necessarily the prominent health needs that will be focused on through a collective effort across the community. Even communities with adequate funding find it necessary to identify priorities that they plan to address. A needs assessment is usually not needed when there is a clear understanding of the community's needs or when there is a priority health need that requires immediate action, such as a COVID-19 response.

Data Sources

There are many data sources available to explore the health of a community and assess what may be the biggest drivers for poor health outcomes. This means that there will be a lot of data to identify, evaluate, and understand. Health needs are often very complex and interconnected. For example, maintaining a healthy weight requires access to healthy foods and safe and accessible venues to engage in physical activity. This can include farmers' markets, bike paths, and walking trails. Maintaining a healthy weight is also about the affordability of foods and the knowledge to prepare healthy meals.

There are multiple sources for health data and multiple types of data. Data can be identified as either quantitative or qualitative data. **Quantitative data** is typically used to describe numbers or statistics that are collected. This could include statistics collected by a local health department, such as the number of syphilis cases. Local health departments report data to a state health department to help identify trends and patterns within the larger community. US territories, freely associated states, and the District of Columbia also have their own health department and collect this type of data. In addition, there is data available on morbidity and mortality in each community. **Morbidity** refers to the quality of life for an individual. It captures information such as the kinds of chronic health conditions prevalent in a community. The term **comorbidities** is used to describe when an individual has multiple chronic health conditions. For example, an individual may be diagnosed with asthma and type 2 diabetes. Discharge data from hospitals, the number of patients seen in an ER during a particular time period, and the number of vaccines distributed among healthcare providers are all examples of quantitative data that can be explored as part of a CHA. Quantitative data can also be collected through surveys. A survey may be used to solicit feedback on existing medical care services for breast cancer screenings. For example, feedback on accessibility and availability of services may be helpful when trying to identify if these are barriers for seeking mammograms. This can be done with a paper survey that is distributed to individuals, an electronic survey delivered over email, or through a phone survey where community members are contacted and asked questions. Qualitative data can also be collected through a windshield tour. A **windshield tour** is essentially when a community is viewed through the windshield of a bus or car and observations are made about community assets and needs.

Activity 3.1: Discussion

Medical schools often include windshield tours as a part of the training for future physicians. This tour, often conducted by riding in a bus, van, or car, is an opportunity to observe the neighborhoods where their future patients live, work, pray, and play. The aim of these tours is for the students to get a deeper understanding of the social determinants of health their patients face.

1. Why do you think a windshield tour is a necessary addition to medical school training?
2. What specific parts of a community do you think the tour should include? Defend your response.

Qualitative data is data that is generally not expressed in statistical information, rather it is data that is expressed in the form of text, images, and audio recordings. For example, a survey may solicit suggestions from community members for locations to install bike racks. The survey could include preidentified street intersections. However, that may result in a very long list yet miss other types of potential locations that community members want to specify in their response. Therefore, including an open-ended question may be helpful to solicit a variety of ideas. Qualitative data can also be captured from interviews or focus groups. Individual interviews or focus groups with youth may offer valuable insight on bullying in schools.

Generally, it is more cumbersome to solicit, collect, and analyze qualitative data than quantitative data. However, qualitative data offers insight that may not be captured in statistics alone. Both types of data are important and necessary to gather, interpret, and analyze to understand drivers of health outcomes, health needs, and opportunities for improvement.

Analyzing Data

Ensuring success in developing programs, policies, and services is guided by the use of evidence-based interventions and best practices. **Evidence-based interventions** are programs, policies, and services that have been proven to be effective. The research on evidence-based interventions demonstrates that when implemented with specific parameters, intended health outcomes are achieved. One helpful tool in identifying what evidence-based interventions exist and how a community (specifically cities and states) compares to others across the country is the Healthy People website.

There are multiple health topics listed on the Healthy People website, though the list is not exhaustive. There may be other health topics that come up for a community and that is ok! This website captures the most common needs and health concerns in the United States, listed as goals and objectives for the nation. The information provided for an objective is incredibly valuable. Baseline data reveals the current average statistic that has been identified for the United States. However, individual communities may experience varying statistics. Baseline data is meant to offer a comparison point and

---

Activity 3.2: Practice your Skills

Let's explore the objectives of Healthy People 2030. You can access Healthy People 2030 at: https://health.gov/healthypeople.

- First, go to the center of the page and select *"Browse objectives by topic."*
- Pick a health topic. For example, you may select "cancer."
    - Note: Search options by Health Behaviors, Populations, Settings and Systems, and Social Determinants of Health are also available.
- Then, review the *goal* listed at the top of the page.
- Next, review the *content* about why this is an important topic to address.
- Finally, select an *objective* that interests you. For the objective, review the *baseline data* that exists and the *recommended target* for each objective.

Table 3.1 Limitations for Addressing Health Concerns

Time Limitations	Resource Limitations	Capacity Limitations
Limited number of hours	Limited funds	Skills and ability of staff
Competing needs	Limited supplies	Skills and ability of volunteers
Volunteers vs paid staff	Limited support	Number of staff

to indicate the reference point from where a goal will be developed. The recommended targets to achieve each goal are listed as objectives.

Limitations

Before developing interventions, it is important to identify the health needs facing a community. The list of health needs in any community can be extensive and complex. In an ideal scenario, each health need is addressed and health outcomes are improved for each member of the community. In reality, there are multiple limitations. These include, but are not limited to, time, resources, and the capacity for any community to make sustainable changes. As indicated in Table 3.1, there may be a limited number of staff and volunteers dedicated to improving health outcomes. This impacts the number of topics that can be addressed and the speed at which interventions are developed or revised.

Addressing social determinants of health may also expose competing needs that each require attention, which means that it may not be possible to give the necessary attention to each topic. Furthermore, there are limitations in funds, supplies, and support. Historically public health has been underfunded (Trust for America's Health, 2022). Often communities rely on time-limited grant funds that require interventions to be completed in a one-, three-, or five-year plan. While that may be helpful in the short term, there may be long-term needs that may go unaddressed with this type of approach. There may be a need for supplies for a program. For example, suppose a community identifies a need for increased access to mammogram screening in a remote area of a town. The community wants to invest in a mobile van to bring mammograms to the community. However, the cost may be a barrier to successfully executing this intervention. The town may not have available funds to dedicate to the project. The volunteers may not be familiar with grant writing and lack confidence in applying for funding. The staff may be assigned to work on multiple projects as part of their role and don't have the capacity to draft a grant application in less than two weeks as it is common for grants to be announced with a deadline within three to four weeks. All of these limitations are very realistic and can impact the number of interventions that can be pursued at a given time in a community. Therefore, it is important to be strategic in identifying and addressing health needs to work toward improving health outcomes.

Community Engagement

The purpose of a CHA is to assess the needs of a community with the intention to develop a plan to address those needs. Including members of the community is important in this work because they have insights and perspectives as someone

Eight Areas of Responsibility for CHES® and MCHES®

Conducting needs assessments and coordinating efforts in developing interventions align with the following Areas of Responsibility for CHES® and MCHES®:

Area I: Assessment of Needs and Capacity

This area includes four competencies and 25 sub-competencies for assessing the needs of communities (National Commission for Health and Education Credentialing, Inc. [NCHEC], 2020). This includes an inventory of existing resources and gaps. Data identification, review, and analysis are also included in this area (NCHEC, 2020). Ultimately, the aim is to identify possible next steps based on the assessment.

Area II: Planning

This area includes four competencies and 19 sub-competencies for planning meaningful interventions in communities (NCHEC, 2020). This includes identifying and engaging members of the community to include members of the community, partner organizations, and others who have a vested interest in the community – often referred to as stakeholders (NCHEC, 2020). This group of individuals works together to identify the priority needs to be addressed and the strategies that will be used.

To learn more about the Areas of Responsibility, please visit: https://www.nchec.org.

SIDEBAR: DID YOU KNOW?

The term *stakeholders* is not a preferred term by the CDC because it can "reflect a power differential between groups and has a violent connotation for some tribes and tribal members. It also groups all parties into one term, despite potential differences in the way they are engaged or interact with a project or activity" (Centers for Disease Control and Prevention [CDC], 2022, para. 35). Therefore, the CDC recommends using language more specific to the role that individuals may have, such as community member or client (2022). Another option is to use language that describes the individuals or group as those who have been impacted or affected, such as community impacted (CDC, 2022). Using language that is inclusive and specific when working with community members is an important part of trust building and relationships.

To learn more about this and other terms that are not the preferred term, please visit: https://www.cdc.gov/health-communication/Preferred_Terms.html.

who lives, works, prays, and plays in that community. Their justification for being involved is often deep and profound. They want their community to thrive and be a place that values and promotes health. Some community members may already be engaged in activities or organizations that address health needs in their community, which is an added benefit for their participation.

Needs Assessments and Planning Models

Once the group of partners has been assembled, the next step is to select a needs assessment and/or a program planning model or framework. Selecting a model or framework determines the route that the group will travel to reach the vision that they have identified.

There are several options of models available to guide the process of conducting a comprehensive needs assessment

SIDEBAR: DID YOU KNOW?

There are many models and frameworks to guide a needs assessment. Many of them share common elements such as:

- Being strategic in approaching the work with a plan,
- Collaborating with and engaging multiple members and organizations in the community,
- Using multiple strategies to collect data to assess the health needs of the community, and
- Identifying the priority health needs (CDC, 2015).

To learn more about other needs assessment and planning models and frameworks, please visit: https://www.cdc.gov/publichealthgateway/index.html and search for *community health assessment and planning.*

for communities to choose from. This chapter will review three models: MAPP, CHANGE, and the PRECEDE-PROCEED.

MAPP Model

The National Association of County and City Health Officials (NACCHO) introduced the **Mobilizing for Action through Planning and Partnerships model (MAPP)** in 1997 as a guide to working with communities to "provide structured guidance that would result in an effective strategic planning process that would be relevant to public health agencies and the communities they serve" (2013, p. 5). The earliest version was developed in 1991 and revised multiple times. Since 2020 NACCHO has been revising and updating the MAPP planning tool again, and released a MAPP 2.0 in July 2023.

MAPP and MAPP 2.0

MAPP and MAPP 2.0 have been included in the book intentionally. The release of MAPP 2.0 occurred while the book was being written in 2023, and it may take time for communities to adopt MAPP 2.0. Therefore, MAPP may be more familiar to some communities.

The MAPP Model includes six phases, as indicated in Table 3.2. Each of the iterative phases is used to strategically solicit guidance and input from multiple community members, partners, and stakeholders. In the first phase, a partnership is formed with the intention of improving health outcomes for a community. These partnerships are composed of community members, partnering organizations, and other stakeholders. Additional stakeholders could include funders or elected officials. The partnership needs to include participants who represent the diverse interests of the community. In addition, since community members are essentially volunteering their time, it is important to consider strategies to ensure their continued engagement. Meeting times and locations can impact the ability of community members to participate. Some volunteers may find that during the process, they have competing commitments and may need to step away, so a partnership may be fluid in membership as some volunteers step back and others may step in. A partnering organization may build participation in the partnership as part of an employee's (or employees') job responsibility, therefore paying them to participate.

Table 3.2 MAPP Model Phases

Phase	Name of Phase	Explanation of Phase
Phase 1	Organize for success/ partnership development	In this phase, a partnership of community members, partners, and interested individuals come together for a common purpose
Phase 2	Visioning	In this phase, partnership participants come together to identify a vision and initial plan
Phase 3	Four MAPP assessments	In this phase, four assessments review and evaluate the current health status of the community, factors that may be responsible for health needs, gaps in care, and opportunities to address
Phase 4	Identify strategic issues	In this phase, partnership participants identify key issues to address in pursuit of achieving the vision identified
Phase 5	Formulate goals and strategies	In this phase, partnership participants identify health outcome goals and the steps to take toward achieving the goals
Phase 6	Action cycle	In this phase, programs, policies, and services are developed or revised. In addition, evaluations are completed to determine if the interventions improved health outcomes and addressed community needs

Note: Adapted from "Introduction" by NACCHO, 2013, p. 4. Retrieved from https://www.oregon.gov/oha/HPA/dsi-tc/CHACHPTechnicalAssistance/MAPP-Handboook.pdf

The second phase is an opportunity for the group to identify their common purpose and vision. Developing a vision involves identifying the inspiration for addressing a complex set of ideas to improve health outcomes. An example of a vision may be listed as, "We are a thriving community where everyone has access to fresh foods and engages in physical activity daily." While the vision statement is something that the partnership will strive to attain, it will take a long time and extensive effort to achieve. Nonetheless, a vision guides the overall work of the partnership throughout this process.

The third phase of the MAPP Model is composed of four assessments. Completing these four assessments provides a rich explanation of the current health status of a community and identifies opportunities for improvement for the partnership to consider. It also provides an opportunity to assess the resources and services already in place that could be enhanced or modified as part of the goal setting in phase five. The assessments in phase three include:

1. The Community Health Status Assessment
2. The Community Themes and Strengths Assessment
3. The Local Public Health System Assessment

The Forces of Change Assessment
The Community Health Status Assessment is a review of quantitative data available to evaluate the overall health of a community (NACCHO, 2013). There may be trends that are identified in the data analysis that demonstrate significant and specific health

outcomes that need attention. The Community Themes and Strengths Assessment is an opportunity to review the resources that are available. These resources are often referred to as assets, as resources are considered valuable tools and services that are available. A distinct feature of the MAPP Model is the third assessment – an assessment of the local public health system. This is an opportunity to review the capacity and opportunities that exist for the local public health system. The public health system can include the local hospital(s), clinic(s), and medical provider(s), as well as other sectors such as media, businesses, and faith-based communities. It is important to evaluate what part of the system may benefit from additional resources, such as staffing or materials, to aid in improving health outcomes. Finally, the Forces of Change Assessment is an evaluation of the context of the community. For example, are there things happening that may contribute to health needs? Perhaps there are multiple construction projects in the community that may be causing an increase in pollutants in the air or the community is recovering from a category 5 hurricane that destroyed much of the local parks when trees were uprooted. Completing each of these four assessments provides a comprehensive review of the needs, resources, and opportunities in the community. It is also what makes the MAPP Model an intense and complex undertaking. So, while there are benefits to knowing this detailed information, it can be a significant amount of work to complete each assessment and review the results.

The fourth phase of the MAPP Model provides the opportunity to identify the key issues contributing to poor health outcomes. There may be an extensive list of key issues, so the vision that was developed initially in the model process is instrumental in helping to determine goals and action steps. The goals and action steps are identified in the fifth phase. Finally, in the sixth phase, the action steps that were identified are completed. This phase can take several

---

SIDEBAR: DID YOU KNOW?

Hospitals are required to conduct community health needs assessments per the Affordable Care Act that was enacted in March 2010. The requirement is connected to their IRS standing as a 501(C)3 organization and mandates that the assessment be completed and made available to the public. The needs assessment needs to define the community and identify significant health needs of the community. Specifically, the health needs must "include requisites for the improvement or maintenance of health status both in the community at large and in particular parts of the community, such as particular neighborhoods or populations experiencing health disparities" (Internal Revenue Service [IRS], 2022, para. 13). Needs may include access to care, illness prevention, and factors that may negatively impact health outcomes. Hospitals are expected to identify the priority health needs by considering the following aspects:

- Toll of the health needs in the community,
- Evidence-based or promising practices to address the health needs,
- Health disparities associated with the health needs, and
- Community buy-in or support for addressing the health need (IRS, 2022).

Just as in the case of a CHA, a hospital may also need to decide not to address a health need because of a lack of resources or capacity. Furthermore, a hospital may recognize that there may already be efforts underway in the community to address the need (IRS, 2022).

years to complete since action steps may span over a large period of time. In addition to implementing the action steps, this phase includes evaluation of the interventions to determine their effectiveness in achieving the goals identified.

According to NACCHO (2013), a community may find that some of these assessments are better suited to be done in combination with one another as opposed to separately. Furthermore, communities may find it more helpful to complete the assessments in a different order to better understand the community. Some partnership members may find it helpful to brainstorm the Forces of Change before identifying the Community Themes and Strengths as some of these may be more apparent after exploring the changes happening in a community.

MAPP Model 2.0

NACCHO conducted an evaluation of MAPP to determine its effectiveness in supporting communities in completing needs assessments and identifying a plan for improving health outcomes. By the end of the evaluation period in 2019, several opportunities for enhancement in the model were identified, including, but limited to, health equity and community engagement (NACCHO, 2023b). Feedback also included an ability for the model to be revised to meet community needs and support ongoing community engagement (NACCHO, 2023b). In July 2023, MAPP 2.0 (as shown in Figure 3.1) was released.

MAPP 2.0 has similarities to MAPP, including multiple community assessments. However, there are only three phases in MAPP 2.0 compared to six phases in MAPP. Phase 1 is focused on establishing the foundation of the multiyear effort of conducting

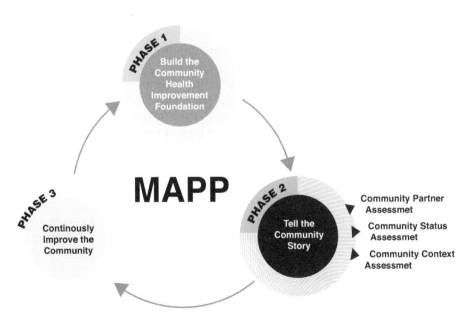

Figure 3.1 MAPP 2.0 Model

Source: Reprinted from Mobilizing for Action Through Planning and Partnerships MAPP 2.0 User's Handbook (p. 4), 2023, National Association of County and City Health Officials (NACCHO). Reprinted with permission.

Table 3.3 MAPP 2.0 Model Phases

Phase	Name of Phase	Explanation of Phase
Phase 1	Build the community health improvement foundation	This phase includes relationship building, a review of available resources, the identification of goals, and a shared agreement on using the MAPP 2.0 model
Phase 2	Tell the community story	This phase includes three primary assessments: a Community Partners Assessment, a Community Status Assessment, and a Community Context Assessment
Phase 3	Continuously improve the community	This phase includes a focus on social determinants of health and health equity by identifying opportunities for improvement on a small scale to demonstrate effectiveness before broader implementation occurs

Note: Adapted from Intro to MAPP 2.0 by NACCHO, n.d. Retrieved from https://www.naccho.org/uploads/card-images/public-health-infrastructure-and-systems/MAPP-2.0-Launch-V3.pdf

a needs assessment. This phase includes identifying partners and collaborators in the community and reviewing available resources. The group will establish a shared vision and identify goals as part of a shared agreement (NACCHO, n.d.). Phase 2 includes multiple assessments to determine the capacity of partners, the health needs of the community, and the context of the data. There are three assessments to accomplish this. The Community Partners Assessment is an opportunity for collaborating community partners to review their own practices and capacity to assist in addressing health inequities (NACCHO, n.d.). The Community Status Assessment is a review of the quantitative data about the health needs in a community and the factors that impact health outcomes (NACCHO, n.d.). Finally, the Community Context Assessment captures qualitative data about the health needs in a community and the perspectives of community members (NACCHO, n.d.). Phase 3 of MAPP 2.0 includes intentional actions in the community to address health inequities collaboratively and logically through small-scale interventions that address social determinants of health and root causes of health inequity (NACCHO, n.d.). In addition to the updated model, communities and HES can access a comprehensive toolkit with sample charts and guidelines to complete each of the phases (Table 3.3).

Activity 3.3: Practice Your Skills

It is vital for HES to know the community and be creative in considering who to invite to a partnership or team working on a CHA. It is so important to think outside of the box. Consider these questions:

1. Who is impacted by the topics that will be identified?
2. Who would care, personally or professionally?
3. What skills can they offer in the process of assessing the needs of the community and helping to create a plan to address the gaps?
   Consider one of the following health needs for the city that you personally either live, work, or study in:

- Obesity
- Diabetes
- Breast Cancer
- Lung Cancer

Then, identify a list of five to seven specific individuals within your specific community representing various agencies, commissions, boards, organizations, neighborhoods, or businesses that would be a potential partner for helping to address this health issue.

1. Who are they?
   - For example, what is their name and background?
2. How did you find them?
   - For example, did you read about something they did recently in a local newspaper or were they referred to you by someone else in the community?
3. What is their role or connection to the community?
   - For example, do they work for an agency in the community or they are an active volunteer for an organization that promotes physical activity?
4. What is their area of expertise?
   - For example, are they an epidemiologist or are they a parent who raised three children in the community and had a family member recently diagnosed with lung cancer?
5. What is your reason for inviting them?
   - For example, do they already volunteer to raise awareness in the community on one of the health needs or do they lead an organization with a mission on one of the topics? Is it because they signed up through a website to indicate their interest in helping?

CHANGE

Another option to guide the community assessment process is **CHANGE, the Community Health Assessment aNd Group Evaluation**. CHANGE uses additional steps, but with similar guiding principles as seen in the MAPP Model. CHANGE is often described as a tool and a planning model in one. It consists of eight steps that include identifying community members to collaborate in assessing various aspects of the community. These steps (as indicated in Table 3.4) include assembling a community team, developing a strategy, reviewing five CHANGE sectors, gathering data, reviewing the data, entering the data, reviewing the consolidated data, and building the Community Action Plan. Each of the subsequent steps of CHANGE ultimately relies on using specific templates developed for communities. The templates enable the team to focus on the data collection and collaboration necessary to conduct a comprehensive assessment. This may help a community conduct a CHA with additional guidance and support.

The first step in using CHANGE is to form a team of 10 to 12 community members. The team identifies how they plan to work together. After reviewing the components of CHANGE, the team may decide to divide the various pieces of the assessment to specific team members. They may decide to have formal meetings and leadership structures or they may decide to be less formal and tackle the various components in subcommittees within the team. CHANGE identifies five sectors to assess in the community. The first is the community at large. This is looking at the community as a whole in terms of assets, gaps, and opportunities. The second sector is the community

Table 3.4 CHANGE Action Steps

Name of Step	Explanation of Step
Assemble the community team	In this step, a team of 10–12 community members is identified and formed to focus on completing the subsequent action steps
Develop team strategy	In this step, the team will decide on how it will operate. Will there be a team lead? How will the tasks be divided up? How often will the team meet? Some teams may find it helpful to formalize their strategy in writing
Review all five CHANGE sectors	In this step, the team will identify the five sectors identified by the CHANGE tool. This includes the community-at-large, community institution/organization, healthcare, school, and worksite. There may be multiple organizations and individuals that will need to be reached out to as part of the assessment process. The team will identify each of these to guide their work
Gather data	In this step, team members are gathering community data from the five sectors
Review data gathered	In this step, team members review the data that was collected and use it to explain the current state of health, assets, gaps, and opportunities
Enter data	In this step, team members use the Excel templates available for CHANGE to analyze the data collected
Review consolidated data	In this step, the Excel templates are reviewed with the data entered in to determine the next steps of the CHANGE process. This step includes completing a summary, developing charts and worksheets to identify the priority health needs and establish goals.
Build the community action plan	In this step, the team will identify the steps of the action plan to achieve the target goals

Note: Adapted from "Action Steps" by Centers for Disease Control and Prevention [CDC], 2021a. Retrieved from https://www.cdc.gov/nccdphp/dnpao/state-local-programs/change-tool/action-steps.html

institutions/organizations. This sector is assessing the various agencies and the services that they provide to the community. This can include social service organizations and academic institutions. The third sector is health care. This includes each of the medical care providers and organizations. Specifically, it can include emergency services, clinics, and preventative care providers. The fourth sector is schools and the fifth sector is work sites. In the third step of CHANGE, team members review each of these sectors to identify a plan for who to contact. Then the team collects the data. It is recommended that at least 13 sites be identified and included in the data collection (CDC, 2021b). Once the data is collected, the team reviews the data and enters it into the provided worksheets and templates provided by CHANGE to identify health needs and priority needs. Once the data is entered into the worksheets and templates, the team is able to analyze the information and identify the desired steps for the Community Action Plan.

Activity 3.4: Discussion
What do you believe are the most important considerations when planning community needs assessments that engage community members? Defend your response.

PRECEDE-PROCEED Model

Since the 1970s public health professionals have been using the **PRECEDE-PROCEED** model in the assessment of communities and development of interventions. Since then, it has been revised multiple times to best guide communities and professionals. This model is rooted in "the disciplines of epidemiology and ecology; the social, behavioral, and educational sciences; and public health administrative and policy studies and experience" (Green, 2023).

The model is composed of eight phases, as indicated in Figure 3.2. The first three phases compose the PRECEDE portion of the model and phases four to eight compose the PROCEED portion. The PRECEDE portion of the model includes three assessments: social assessment, epidemiological assessment, and educational and ecological assessment. In this chapter, these assessments will be explored.

The social assessment in the first phase identifies what the vision is for the quality of life that community members seek. This vision setting drives the rest of the phases. The second phase is an epidemiological assessment of the health factors. This includes morbidity and mortality data that captures what is impacting the health of the community. These are factors that are informed by individual genetics, individual health behaviors, and environmental factors. Environmental factors can include air

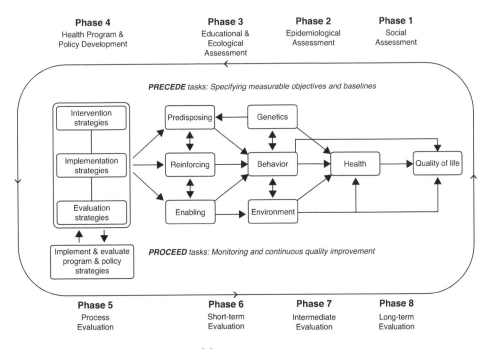

Figure 3.2 PRECEDE-PROCEED Model

Source: Reprinted from Health Program Planning, Implementation, and Evaluation: Creating Behavioral, Environmental, and Policy Change (p. 17), edited by Lawrence W. Green, Andrea Carlson Gielen, Judith M. Ottoson, Darleen V. Peterson, and Marshall W. Kreuter, 2008, Johns Hopkins University Press. Copyright 2008 by Johns Hopkins University Press. Reprinted with permission.

pollution or lead from paint in older homes. The third phase includes an assessment of predisposing, reinforcing, and enabling factors. **Predisposing factors** may raise the risk for specific health conditions. This includes genetics, family history, or age. **Reinforcing factors** are factors that contribute to specific behaviors. For example, at worksites, financial incentives for participating in health promotion activities may encourage individuals to engage in behaviors that they may not typically do. Reinforcing factors can also be negative, such as when someone in a social group consistently provides tobacco products to others so that they are not alone in smoking. Finally, **enabling factors** are factors that support behaviors. For example, a community with sidewalks, bike paths, and walking trails provides opportunities for and encourages physical activity. The opposite can also happen. Communities may not have these elements in place making outdoor cycling, running, and walking less appealing and safe. Reviewing these and similar factors through these three assessments is a comprehensive approach that may or may not be included in the other models and frameworks.

Considerations for Selecting a Model, Framework, or Tool

Since there are several pathways that a community can take in completing a CHA, it is important to consider which model, framework, or tool would work best. Some considerations include:

- Readiness
- Timeline
- Who will participate in partnership or team
- Capacity to conduct data collection
- Confidence in using a specific model, framework, or tool

HES may find it beneficial to review these considerations in their role and with the community members that they work with. Readiness refers to how prepared the community is to start the assessment process. Perhaps the assessment is a requirement that needs to be completed within a specific time period or the capacity of the team is limited and the assessment period is abbreviated. Each assessment model and framework has a focus on collaborative efforts with community members. While CHANGE specified 10–12 team members, the MAPP Model utilizes more members of the community as part of the partnership. In addition to this core group, they will need to collaborate with others in the community. There may be specific times of the year that may work better than others. Consider religious observances, for example. If the upcoming months have multiple days that will impact availability, then the timeline may need to be adjusted or altered. Identifying the core group is also a consideration. Perhaps the core group is missing representation from the diverse aspects of the community being assessed. Before beginning the process, there may need to be some additional recruitment. Who is in the core group and their capacity to complete the recommended steps in a model or framework is also a valuable consideration. There may be interest in receiving training about the model or framework before beginning the process. This may be a valuable investment in the process to ensure success.

Some communities may find that specific elements from various models, frameworks, and tools work best for them. That is ok! The MAPP Handbook explains that "[c]ommunities with little assessment and planning experience may decide to try a portion of the process before committing to the entire process" (NACCHO, 2013). Communities and the HES that work alongside them will know best how to approach the work, when to pause and reflect, and when to proceed. Setting aside for these reflections is a critical component of this work.

SIDEBAR: DID YOU KNOW?

A valuable resource of detailed explanations and guidance for communities and HES is the Community Toolbox. Across 46 chapters, this online resource hosts slides, videos, and worksheets to aid in needs assessments, coalition building, developing and evaluating interventions, and more.

Please visit: https://ctb.ku.edu/en to explore this resource.

Concepts in Action 3.1

Background: Tasha (she/her) is employed at the local hospital. She has been tasked with developing programs to improve population health. One of her main responsibilities is to solicit feedback from the community on the recent CHA that the hospital completed to identify the priority health needs.

Today Tasha is meeting with a group of about 25 community members. Per the IRS guidelines for hospitals in conducting a CHA, the group is composed of representation from the local health department and "members of medically underserved, low-income, and minority populations in the community served by the hospital facility, or individuals or organizations serving or representing the interests of these populations" (IRS, 2022, para. 18). Each participant in the meeting has reviewed the preliminary draft developed by the hospital and is prepared to share their ideas and recommendations for which health needs are most urgent, pressing, and need intentional efforts over the next three to five years. Soon into the meeting, Tasha realizes that there is much disagreement among the participants and the conversation is getting heated as individuals are starting to talk over each other to convey their perspective. Tasha considers three strategies to help the group share their thoughts on the priority health needs in an effective way. These include brainstorming, conducting and nominal group activity, and voting.

Identifying Priorities

Once health needs are identified, narrowing the focus of what to address can be an exciting yet daunting process. This process begins with reviewing the collected health data about a community, which can often be quite overwhelming. Each of the health needs that are identified in a CHA is important to the individuals and the community members who have been impacted by them. So, when the decision has to be made to prioritize the health needs, it can be a difficult task.

There are two important factors that can aid in this process. First, it is critical that a diverse representation of community members and organizations has an opportunity to review the list of health needs to address. These are the individuals who live, work, pray, and play in the community and their insight on the needs is critical to explaining the interconnectedness, any invisible barriers, and historical context. These individuals want to have their community be the best one possible and so their commitment to this process needs to be validated and supported. The second factor is that each of them will bring with them lived experiences, personally and/or professionally, and they will want to process these. That means that creating opportunities for a facilitated conversation that promotes communication is essential. This means that it may take longer than expected to hear from all individuals. So, longer meetings or multiple meetings may be necessary to ensure this. It is not uncommon for this process to take longer than expected. However, while it may take longer it should also be well facilitated. This ensures a productive discussion occurs with a focus on identifying and agreeing upon priorities. It also aids in creating a space where individuals feel valued and appreciated for their insight.

There are a few strategies that are helpful in a facilitated discussion to identify priority needs. These include brainstorming, conducting and nominal group activity, and voting. Brainstorming is an intentional opportunity to share ideas and thoughts. In this case, it would be to capture ideas on which of the health needs they believe should be a priority health need. This may be done by asking a large group for ideas and capturing them in writing. It may be helpful to divide the group into smaller groups to brainstorm and then share their ideas with the larger group. Another option is to ask participants to identify their ideas on a worksheet or piece of paper prior to the meeting (or at the start of the meeting) and then giving each person an opportunity to share their ideas. Depending on the size of the group, the amount of time dedicated to the meeting, and the comfort of the facilitator each of these may be used as part of the brainstorming session.

After soliciting ideas and feedback on the identified health needs, it may be useful to conduct a nominal group activity. For example, if Tasha (the HES introduced in the *Concepts in Action*) were to use this strategy then she would review the list captured in the brainstorming session. Let's assume that the group reviewed the data and was able to identify 15 topics that they believe are priority needs. Perhaps some of these overlap with each other and the group agrees that there are 12 topics. The reality is that each topic would have multiple action steps and interventions, so it would not be possible to have 12 priority topics. The group agrees that they have the capacity and resources to focus on four priority topics. This means that Tasha needs to aid the group in identifying which four health needs they agree on. A nominal group activity would then include giving the group the opportunity to cast a vote for four of the 12 topics. After the first round, this may narrow the list to nine topics. Tasha opens the conversation back up for further discussion. It may be that the group breaks and re-convenes at another time to narrow the list from nine to four. When the group is ready to resume, Tasha will re-engage with the participants to solicit their vote with the intention of identifying four topics out of the nine that the group agrees are priority topics. This example demonstrates that the group works together to identify the priority needs.

Another strategy to consider is to offer limited voting. Tasha may be meeting with the participants in person and have posted pieces of paper around the room. Each piece of paper lists one of the 12 topics. Each participant is given four stickers and after discussing the topics they place their sticker on four of the topics. The four topics that have the most stickers on them are the priority health needs.

Activity 3.5: Discussion

After reviewing *Concept in Action 3.1*, how would you respond to each of the following questions?

1. Which of the described strategies would you recommend to Tasha? Defend your recommendation.
2. Are there other strategies that you would recommend that Tasha consider? Describe the strategy.

Community Health Improvement Plans

In the CHANGE tool and planning model, the end result is the development of a Community Action Plan. Another commonly used term to describe this is a **Community Health Improvement Plan,** sometimes referred to as a CHIP. A CHIP is a detailed plan with identified goals, objectives, and action steps. Typically, a CHIP will indicate the specific individuals or organizations that will take a leading role for specific objectives. It is usually the end product of a needs assessment process and is referred to throughout the planning process and in evaluation efforts.

Activity 3.6: Practice Your Skills

This is a brief example of demographic data collected as part of a CHA for a fictional small town on the east coast. Review the information presented and consider your responses to the discussion questions.

Community Demographics

Median Age: (U.S. Census, 2019)
   U.S.: 38.1
   State: 36
   Town: 33.2

Life Expectancy:
   U.S.: 78.8
   State: 77
   Town: 72

Average Family Size: (U.S. Census, 2021)
   U.S.: 3.1
   State: 4.2
   Town: 4.7

1. What stands out to you about the data? Do you notice any trends?
2. Why would this information be important to include in a CHA?
3. What do you think about *how* the information was presented? Is there a better way to display the information?

Many communities and hospitals make their CHA documents readily available online. Conduct an internet search for a CHA in your own state or region. You may want to look for multiple examples to compare urban and rural communities. You can also search for Community Health Assessments at: https://www.naccho.org/. After reviewing the CHA, consider the same discussion questions.

Summary

- The purpose of conducting needs assessments in communities is to identify what the current health status is in a community and where opportunity exists for improvement.
- There are several models, frameworks, and tools available for a community health needs assessment. While there are many similarities between them, there are also differences. It is important to determine which strategy works best for the team dedicated to the work.
- There are many ways to identify priority topics. It is important to include community input in this process. Strategies such as brainstorming, using a nominal group activity, and voting can aid in reaching consensus.
- Assessment activities may take a few months to over a year to complete. This extensive process is designed to ultimately design a community health improvement plan. However, not all of the health needs that are identified can be included in CHIP due to limitations in staffing, capacity, and resources. These limitations impact population health because there will be health needs that do not receive focused efforts.

Web Resources

- **Community Tool Box**

  https://ctb.ku.edu/en

  This resource from the Center for Community Health and Development at the University of Kansas was developed to help community members and leaders to increase their capacity in supporting community health improvement efforts. Topics range from community needs assessments to leading meetings. Each topic covered includes slides, videos, and links to examples across the country.

- **NACCHO**

  https://www.naccho.org/

  The National Association of County and City Health Officials (NACCHO) supports about 3,000 local and tribal health departments with technical assistance, policy development, and research (2023a). Their website provides success stories, including examples of CHAs and CHIPs. To learn more, search for *Community Health Assessment* and *CHIP*.

- **State & Territorial Health Department Websites**

  https://www.cdc.gov/publichealthgateway/healthdirectories/healthdepartments.html

  To learn more about the services and programs available at each state, territory, and freely associated state, please review this website for a link to each available website.

References

Centers for Disease Control and Prevention. (2015). *Assessment & Planning Models, Frame works & Tools*. Center for State, Tribal, Local, and Territorial Support. https://www.cdc.gov/publichealthgateway/cha/assessment.html

Centers for Disease Control and Prevention. (2021a). *Action Steps*. Division of Nutrition, Physical Activity, and Obesity. https://www.cdc.gov/nccdphp/dnpao/state-local-programs/change-tool/action-steps.html

Centers for Disease Control and Prevention. (2021b). *Action Step 4: Gather Data*. Division of Nutrition, Physical Activity, and Obesity. https://www.cdc.gov/nccdphp/dnpao/state-local-programs/change-tool/actionstep4.html

Centers for Disease Control and Prevention. (2022). *Preferred Terms for Select Population Groups & Communities*. https://www.cdc.gov/healthcommunication/Preferred_Terms.html

Internal Revenue Service. (2022). *Community Health Needs Assessment for Charitable Hospital Organizations - Section 501(r)(3)*. https://www.irs.gov/charities-non-profits/community-health-needs-assessment-for-charitable-hospital-organizations-section-501r3

Green, L.W., Gielen, A.C., Ottoson, J.M., Peterson, D.V., & Kreuter, M. W. (Ed.). (2008). *Health Program Planning, Implementation, and Evaluation: Creating Behavioral, Environmental, and Policy Change*. Johns Hopkins University Press.

Green, L.W. (2023). *The PRECEDE-PROCEED Model 2022 Edition*. https://www.lgreen.net/precede-proceed-2022-edition

National Association of County and City Health Officials. (n.d.). *Intro to MAPP 2.0*. https://www.naccho.org/uploads/card-images/public-health-infrastructure-and-systems/MAPP-2.0-Launch-V3.pdf

National Association of County and City Health Officials. (2013, September). *Mobilizing for Action through Planning and Partnerships (MAPP) User's Handbook*. https://santarosa.floridahealth.gov/programs-and-services/community-health-planning-and-statistics/_documents/MAPP-Users-Handbook.pdf

National Association of County and City Health Officials. (2023a). *About*. https://www.naccho.org/about

National Association of County and City Health Officials. (2023b). *Mobilizing for Action Through Planning & Partnerships MAPP 2.0 User's Handbook*. https://toolbox.naccho.org/pages/tool-view.html?id=6012

National Commission for Health and Education Credentialing, Inc. (2020). *Areas of Responsibility, Competencies and Sub-competencies for Health Education Specialist Practice Analysis II 2020 (HESPA II 2020)*. https://assets.speakcdn.com/assets/2251/hespa_competencies_and_sub-competencies_052020.pdf

Trust for America's Health. (2022, July). *The Impact of Chronic Underfunding on America's Public Health System: Trends, Risk, and Recommendations, 2022*. https://www.tfah.org/wp-content/uploads/2022/07/2022PublicHealthFundingFINAL.pdf

CHAPTER 4

Evaluating Programs: Measuring for Success

Learning Objectives

After reading this chapter, learners will be able to:

- ■ Describe the importance of evaluation in health education and promotion program delivery
- ■ Differentiate between types of evaluation
- ■ Describe the process of writing and disseminating evaluation reports
- ■ Explain strategies to ensure program evaluation activities are appropriate and effective

Keywords

- ■ Accuracy Standards
- ■ Baseline Data
- ■ Evaluation Standards
- ■ External Evaluator
- ■ Feasibility Standards
- ■ Formative Evaluation
- ■ Goals
- ■ Impact Evaluation
- ■ Internal Evaluator
- ■ National Standards for Culturally and Linguistically Appropriate Services (CLAS)
- ■ Objectives
- ■ Outcome Evaluation
- ■ Process Evaluation
- ■ Propriety Standards
- ■ Summative Evaluation
- ■ Target Population
- ■ Utility Standards

DOI: 10.4324/9781003504320-4

Self-Reflection Questions

Take a moment and think about an evaluation you participated in. Perhaps you completed an evaluation of a professor or responded to a satisfaction survey after a medical appointment. Then reflect on these questions about the evaluation you completed:

1. What was the purpose of the evaluation or survey?
2. Who will likely read the results?
3. How might the results be used? Did this influence what you shared in your evaluation?

The purpose of any health promotion program or intervention is to improve health outcomes. This might include an increase in the uptake of healthy behaviors (such as an increase in physical activity) and a decrease in unhealthy behaviors (such as smoking less or stopping smoking). Some interventions or programs can be relatively easy to implement over a short period of time, while others may be implemented over months and years. HES are typically spending limited time and other valuable resources on implementing health interventions or programs, and when the desired outcomes of these are achieved they need to be identified and documented. For example, by the end of the 15-week intervention, do the participants report being more physically active? Did the rate of obesity among the group of participants decrease? Has there been any improvement in the desired health outcome? Funders, elected officials, and other invested partners will want to know if the desired results were achieved and to what extent. Fortunately, there are many tools, resources, and techniques to effectively conduct health promotion program evaluations. HES can play multiple roles in the program evaluation process. For example, they may choose the type of evaluation design, evaluation measures that will be a part of an intervention, identify the type of data collected, interpret and analyze the data, draft findings, develop a final report, and choose a communication strategy or strategies to share the evaluation results. In this chapter, the purpose and types of evaluation will be discussed.

Purpose of Evaluation

Typically, evaluations are considered simply to identify if the objectives and the goal were met or not met. **Goals** and **objectives** for interventions and programs guide and inform how and why an intervention or program is even being implemented. It is essential to consider what the overall purpose of the intervention is. For example, the goal may be that adult community members are all engaging in physical activity (as indicated in Table 4.1).

The goal does not describe what type of physical activity or for how long. It also does not share how this would be measured. These details are typically provided in an objective. Objectives are more specific and give details as to how the goal will be achieved. For example, if the goal is for residents to feel valued and respected, an objective could be that monthly sessions are available for networking opportunities.

Table 4.1 Examples of Goals and Objectives

Goal	Objective Example
Adults in the community regularly engage in physical during the week	By December 31, 2028, 50% of the adults in the community will report getting at least 30 minutes of exercise at least 5 days per week
Each resident feels valued and respected	By March 1, 2027, monthly networking programs will be in place to welcome new residents to the facility

Goal and Objectives

The topic of developing goals and objectives is further explored in Chapter 5. This includes covering the different types of objectives, such as process, impact, and outcome objectives.

Program evaluations can be a valuable tool in providing insight on the coordination of the logistics of the intervention or program. Specifically, questions about the delivery of the intervention or program can be identified with one or more of the following questions:

1. Did the intervention reach the intended members of the community? Why or why not?
2. Did the intervention reach members beyond the community that were not targeted? If yes, which community was reached?
3. Were the goals and objectives of the intervention or program met?
4. Were there any unintended or unexpected outcomes?
5. Was the intervention or program delivered as designed? If not, what modifications were made and why?
6. What lessons were learned about the intervention or program delivery or implementation?
7. What were the challenges and barriers in the implementation process?
8. Was the intervention accepted and adopted within the community? Why or why not?
9. How can the intervention be improved?
10. Were there components of the intervention that worked better than others? If so, what were they and what made them more effective?

It is also important to consider the satisfaction of the participants who were involved in the intervention or program. This can be evaluated with questions such as:

1. Were the participants satisfied with the intervention or program? What worked and what could have been better from their perspective?
2. Would the participants recommend participating in this intervention or program to a friend?

Feedback about the intervention or program can also provide insight for the planning and implementation of future interventions and programs. Questions to assess this can include:

1. Can the intervention be replicated or would modifications be necessary? Why?
2. Is the intervention sustainable? If yes, what is necessary to ensure this happens?
3. Can the results be used as a rationale for continuing the program or starting a new program?
4. Should a previous funder award funds to continue the intervention? Why or why not?

Activity 4.1: Discussion

Consider the following questions about evaluations:

1. After reviewing the list of questions that can be asked in an evaluation about the delivery of an intervention or program, what additional insight can an evaluation provide? What questions can be asked to garner this information?
2. When do you think planning for evaluation needs to begin?
3. Who is responsible for conducting program evaluation?

Planning for Evaluation

To ensure that evaluations occur as part of the implementation of an intervention or program, they must be included in the planning process. Planning for evaluation is most effective when it occurs in the early stages of intervention design and development. Depending on what is being evaluated, it can be extremely difficult to go back and evaluate something after it has already occurred. For example, if an objective of the intervention or program was to demonstrate an increase in knowledge among community members, then data on that knowledge before the intervention or program was implemented is necessary. The data that is collected before the intervention or program begins is referred to as **baseline data**. Without baseline data, it will be difficult to measure change. Thus, decisions and plans for evaluation must be made before the implementation of an intervention. This means that HES must incorporate discussions on evaluation during the assessment and planning process phases.

During this process, HES must also keep in mind that there may be several

> **SIDEBAR: DID YOU KNOW?**
>
> If you are interested in this topic, then you may be interested in a career in evaluation. This means that you can lead the efforts in developing evaluation plans for interventions and programs and analyze the data to identify important information to disseminate to all of the interested parties.
>
> The American Evaluation Association is a professional association to support program evaluators with conferences, publications, evaluation tools, training opportunities, and policy updates. To learn more about the Association and the many benefits of membership for evaluation professionals, please visit: https://www.eval.org.

individuals and organizations who will be interested in learning the outcomes of a program. This can include project staff, program managers, community partners, members of the **target population** (the individuals or groups of people for which an intervention or program is intended), elected officials, and funders. Results may be used to garner continued support for the intervention and provide justification for future funding. They may also be disseminated to the broader scientific community for research and replication.

Conducting the Evaluation

Another important decision that needs to be made early in the process is who will be responsible for conducting the evaluation. Will it be an internal person, such as a member of the implementation team, a program supervisor, another staff person, an agency manager or director, or an outside contractor? There are benefits and challenges to selecting an **internal evaluator** versus an **external evaluator** (as indicated in Table 4.2). Benefits of using an internal evaluator include assigning the responsibility to a staff member who is already familiar with the project goal and objectives. They will typically be able to assume this responsibility as part of their existing duties. An internal evaluator will also generally have existing relationships with the project team which may make communication easier and support more frequent updates with the project team. Finally utilizing an internal evaluator is generally less expensive because the individual is already getting paid to be a part of the project, this is just a responsibility that they are tasked with. Challenges for selecting an internal evaluator may include that the person chosen for the role may have a bias toward a favorable evaluation because they are a part of the project team and organization. In addition, they may not be open to new ideas or ways of reviewing the implementation of an intervention or program because they may believe the way that the intervention or program is done is the best and "this is how we have always done it." Finally, assigning the role of an evaluator to someone within an organization or as part of a project team may conflict with the tasks and roles that they already have. There may be limited time available for them to take on an extra task unless this is something that has been written into an existing job description for their role.

The benefits of hiring an external evaluator include less chance for bias, less chance for conflicts with other responsibilities that the project staff members may not have,

Table 4.2 Benefits and Challenges of an Internal versus External Evaluator

Benefits of an Internal Evaluator	Benefits of an External Evaluator
■ Existing knowledge	■ Objectivity and less bias
■ Time can be dedicated to the project	■ Limited schedule conflicts
■ Maintain close ties to project team	■ New ideas and perspectives
■ Generally less expensive	
Challenges of an Internal Evaluator	**Challenges of an External Evaluator**
■ Personal or organizational bias	■ Lack of familiarity
■ May not be open to new ideas	■ Availability
■ Staff member may not have the time	■ Generally more expensive

and allows for new ideas to be introduced to the evaluation. Selecting an external evaluator may reduce the chance that the evaluator has a personal or professional bias for the success of the program and this may be indicated by their objective perspective. An external evaluator will not typically be aware of existing relationships, challenges, or other dynamics that may play a role in planning for and implementing an intervention or program within the community. This may aid in a comprehensive review of the various components with less or no judgment. Typically, an external evaluator will only support the intervention or program with the evaluation components which allows them to focus just on this aspect, as opposed to an internal evaluator who may or may not have additional job duties. Finally, external evaluators bring with them the experience and knowledge of other interventions and programs and this could be helpful when addressing challenges or barriers that may be discovered in the evaluation process or results. Their knowledge may be helpful to a project team that is looking for creative and appropriate solutions.

Challenges of an external evaluator can include the loss of some control over the how and when of the evaluation is completed and it is likely to be more expensive than using an internal evaluator. External evaluators may need time to review and understand the various components of a proposed intervention or program, which can sometimes occur over weeks, months, and years. This may mean that they miss some of the background and justification for why certain decisions were made for the implementation of the intervention or program and what the assumptions were of their impact. Although an external evaluator may not be busy with other tasks of the intervention or program that they were selected to evaluate, they may have other projects that they are working on. This may then impact their availability. This can be frustrating to the project team because the external evaluator may need to miss meetings or have to delay their timeline for sharing their work. An external evaluator will also need to be selected. This may be an extensive process of posting a job description, conducting interviews, and then making an offer. Because cost is an important factor when considering who will conduct the evaluation, including this early in the planning process can help avoid budget shortfalls.

Activity 4.2: Discussion

Imagine you are a health educator employed by a local health department and you have been tasked with implementing a vaping prevention program at a local high school. You are teaching an eight-week curriculum and the school is funding the project. The school board is very interested in the results of the program because if the program is successful then this could result in positive visibility throughout the state. Your supervisor is also very excited about the potential success of the program because the partnership between the local health department and the school system has not always been positive. Consider the following questions and share your thoughts with a peer.

1. For this program, do you think it would be better to have an internal evaluator (such as a school or health department employee) or an external evaluator (perhaps a local professor)?

2. What are some ways the school could reduce bias if using an internal evaluator?
3. What are some questions an external evaluator might ask the health department or you, the health educator, before agreeing to conduct a program evaluation for that agency?

Evaluating Programs

The focus of the next section is only on evaluating health education and promotion programs, also referred to as just programs, and does not address evaluating interventions specifically. There are some significant differences in evaluating interventions, which typically involve a control and a test group, which are beyond the scope of this book. Typically a course on research evaluation or methodology will explore this topic.

Types of Program Evaluation

There are five main types of program evaluation: process evaluation, formative evaluation, impact evaluation, outcome evaluation, and summative evaluation (as indicated in Table 4.3). Each of these types of evaluation considers different measures and data about and from a program, and they each serve a distinct and important role to inform program staff and other interested parties about the successes and missed opportunities of the program. While each evaluation plan to assess programs will differ, most plans utilize all or a combination of the different types of evaluations.

Table 4.3 Types of Evaluation

Evaluation Type	Description
Process	Evaluates how and how well an intervention was implemented. This includes aspects such as if the activities were completed as planned and if any changes were made during implementation. Maintaining a log of implementation challenges or changes made during the program can help inform this type of evaluation.
Formative	Assesses the success and quality of an intervention. This evaluation is conducted throughout the implementation and helps to inform programmatic changes and justify needed updates.
Impact	Evaluates measures of change that occurred as a result of the program. This can include both immediate and long-term changes in behavior, attitudes, knowledge, or the environment.
Outcome	Focuses on medium- and long-term outcomes, such as changes in health status or health indicators. These are typically measured two to five years after an intervention.
Summative	A cumulative process that can include all of the types of evaluation. This evaluation can provide an overview of whether stated goals and objectives were met.

HES use the stated objectives of the intervention to guide the evaluation process. **Process evaluation** refers to how the activities of the program were completed. It is typically conducted at the end of an evaluation. Process evaluation is similar to **formative evaluation**, which measures the success and quality of the actual implementation of the program, from the initial steps to completion. Formative evaluation occurs concurrently with the program and allows for real-time adjustments to maintain or improve quality. Process evaluation might include how many posters were created and distributed, how many hand-washing demonstrations occurred, and how many flu clinics were held. In process evaluation, the concern is not about the impact or effectiveness of the intervention, it is only about how well the activities of the intervention were conducted. Process evaluation is one way HES can document what was done, by whom, and how well it was done. Process evaluations are also important if another agency or organization CDC is interested in replicating the intervention because it provides them with insight on implementation. Therefore, process evaluations need to be objective in reporting on exactly what did and did not actually happen.

An **impact evaluation** measures changes in knowledge, attitudes, and behaviors. For example, what changed in the attitude of the participant as a result of the program? In a follow-up survey three months after the program, are participants reporting an increase in physical activity? Did they report an increase in the number of fruits and vegetables they consume each day? After each session, was there increased knowledge of the risk factors associated with sexual behaviors? Perhaps there was a change in attitude about using birth control. These changes are typically measured at the conclusion of the intervention, but may also be measured over time to capture sustained behavior change. A worksite flu prevention program might evaluate whether individuals report an increase in hand-washing, getting a flu vaccine, and consistently using cough and sneeze etiquette three months, six months, and nine months after the program ended, and if hand sanitizers were installed throughout the building.

An **outcome evaluation** is focused on longer-term changes in health indicators, health outcomes, or disease rates. For example, this may include a decrease in breast cancer or obesity rates. This type of evaluation is frequently linked to evaluating the success of the overall goal of the program. Outcome evaluations can take longer to conduct because the data is gathered and analyzed during the program, after the program, and typically years after the program ended. For example, statistically significant decreases in obesity rates may not be achieved for years after a program. It is not uncommon to collect this data two to five years after a program ends. However, a significant challenge for conducting an outcome evaluation is that HES and the programs that they support and lead may not have the sustained staffing and funding to conduct outcome evaluation months or years after the program ends. In addition, there may be other factors that contribute to changes in health outcomes, such as other interventions or programs, social influences, and policy changes. These additional factors are frequently outside of the control of the HES and the program staff and they can sometimes make it very difficult to show cause and effect. This means an evaluation may not be able to state that program is what caused a change. An example of this is when flu shot uptake increased during the COVID-19 pandemic as many people viewed their susceptibility as being higher. The vaccination rate for adults over the age of 18 increased by 1.8% from the 2019–2020 to the 2020–2021 flu season (Centers for Disease Control and Prevention [CDC], 2021).

Finally, **summative evaluations** encompass all of the types of evaluation. This evaluation can include measures on how effective the program was from the initial planning stages to completion utilizing all of the data collected. HES can decide which evaluation types will be included in the summative evaluation. Finally, a summative evaluation will be included in the final evaluation report typically provided to the funder of the program. The final report typically only includes evaluation findings that are deemed important and significant by the HES, project staff, and invested partners.

Activity 4.3: Practice Your Skills

Access the listing of five reports for the 2013–2018 Fairfax County Community Health Improvement Plan (CHIP) Evaluation at: https://tinyurl.com/4kj2zsns. At the bottom of the webpage, a link is provided for each of the five yearly reports. Please select one and review it.

After reviewing the evaluation report, please share your responses to the following questions about the information provided:

1. Review one priority issue area, such as Healthy and Safe Physical Environments, and identify which *Key Actions* are indicative of a process, formative, impact, outcome, and summative evaluation.
2. For that same priority issue area, how do the measures align with the stated objectives? Will these measures provide the needed information to determine the success of the CHIP?
3. For that same priority issue area, review the *Responsible Parties*. Were internal or external partners responsible for the interventions? Were they also responsible for the evaluation? How do you know?

Fairfax County Community Health Improvement Plan

The Fairfax County Community Health Improvement Plan is further explored in Chapter 5, with a specific focus on assessment, planning, issue prioritization, and community engagement.

CDC Framework for Program Evaluation

Selecting an evaluation type and conducting evaluations can feel like a daunting process. However, there are tools and resources available for HES to be successful. The Centers for Disease Control and Prevention (CDC) developed a framework to be used in the early stages of program planning to conduct program evaluation (CDC, 1999). The framework consists of six steps that work together to inform the development of a comprehensive program evaluation that will serve the many interested parties interested in the results. The steps (as indicated in Figure 4.1) include engaging the stakeholders, describing the program, focusing on an evaluation design, gathering credible evidence, justifying the conclusions, and using the lessons learned from the evaluation and sharing them with others (CDC, 1999).

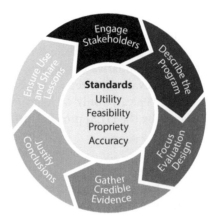

Figure 4.1 Framework for Program Evaluation in Public Health

Note: From Centers for Disease Control and Prevention. (2017). A Framework for Program Evaluation. Retrieved from https://www.cdc.gov/evaluation/framework/index.htm. In the public domain.

Step 1: Engage Stakeholders

Stakeholders are individuals or groups who are invested in the success of the program and the health and well-being of the target population. These are considered the primary audience for an evaluation report. Stakeholders can and should be engaged at all stages of the intervention, from initial planning through final evaluation. Stakeholders can also be called invested partners and collaborators. Examples of ways to engage stakeholders include convening steering or planning committee meetings before, during, and after the intervention; conducting interviews; and capturing any feedback offered by this group.

Engaging Others

The topic of engaging individuals or groups who are invested and interested in the success of a program is further explored in Chapter 5.

Step 2: Describe the Program

A description of the program typically includes the rationale for the program, results of a needs assessment that informed the development of the program, a description of the target audience, objectives and action steps, financial and staffing resources needed, responsible parties for program implementation and evaluation, and the expected benefits to participants and the community.

Step 3: Focus Evaluation Design

HES will decide how to organize the design of the evaluation in this step. Design considerations can include: What tools will be needed to implement and evaluate the intervention? Will the timing of the evaluation align with the implementation? If so, how? Who will be involved in the evaluation process? What is the expected timeline for completing the evaluation? This step includes decisions about how and what data will be collected and analyzed. Consider the evaluation measures that will be used to determine if the objectives of the intervention were met.

Step 4: Gather Credible Evidence

The next step is to collect the data, organize it, and store it in a way that it can be easily accessed. Evidence can be gathered in a number of ways: pre- and post-surveys, only post-surveys, key informant interviews, direct observation, focus groups, and HES and participant self-reports. Data can also be obtained from attendance sheets, test responses, and feedback forms.

Step 5: Justify Conclusions

This step includes using appropriate and scientific data analysis methods to review the collected data and determine what they say about the program. Recommendations for future iterations of the program are also based on the findings. In some cases, the results may be compared to national benchmarks or established norms. In this step, comparisons can be made back to the initial needs assessment, rationale, and goals and objectives of the intervention.

> **SIDEBAR: DID YOU KNOW?**
>
> The Community Toolbox describes several types of data to collect and the methods of data collection in Chapter 37. To learn more, please review the chapter at: https://ctb.ku.edu/en/table-of-contents/evaluate/evaluate-community-interventions.

Step 6: Ensure Use and Share Lessons

The final step of a comprehensive program evaluation includes sharing the results and lessons learned from the evaluation. At the local level, this may be a presentation to the City Council or Board of Health. Other examples of this can include a formal report to a funder, submitting a journal article, drafting a case study, delivering a conference presentation, or other communication strategy. Channels used can include print, social media, and professional conferences.

> **Professional Development**
>
> The responsibility to share and disseminate results and findings with others in the field is discussed in more detail in Chapter 9. This chapter explores how important this is as a part of the professional development of HES.

Activity 4.4: Practice Your Skills

There are many steps involved in program evaluation. To support HES in ensuring that each recommended step is included in their evaluation, they can use CDC Evaluation Planning Tools. Review these three evaluation checklists:

https://www.cdc.gov/tb/programs/evaluation/guide/pdf/evaluation_plan_template.pdf
https://www.cdc.gov/evaluation/steps/step1/Step-1-Checklist-Final.pdf
https://www.cdc.gov/evaluation/steps/step2/Step-2-Checklist-Final.pdf
https://www.cdc.gov/evaluation/steps/step3/Step-3-Checklist-Final.pdf

After reviewing the checklists, imagine you and your peers are collaborating on a health promotion team that has been tasked with implementing a tobacco use prevention program at a local middle and high school. Consider how you might ensure that you have a solid evaluation plan ready.

Evaluation Standards

There are four **evaluation standards** that are incorporated into the CDC's framework for building a comprehensive evaluation process (CDC, 2017). These have also been further defined and explained by the Joint Committee on Standards for Educational Evaluation (2023). Evaluation standards are an important component because incorporating them increases the likelihood that the evaluation will be useful and meaningful to stakeholders (CDC, 2017; Yarbrough et al., 2010). The four standards are utility, feasibility, propriety, and accuracy.

Utility standards are about ensuring that the information that is provided in an evaluation is useful and helpful to the interested parties. In order to improve public health and know that the work of HES and others is impactful, the information contained in an evaluation must be clear, able to be understood, and able to be implemented in future programs to improve outcomes. Considerations when examining the utility of information being presented in an evaluation include who conducted the evaluation, how cultural considerations were integrated, and how the results were utilized.

Feasibility standards are about how practical the evaluation is to complete based on the available resources. Is it possible to do this evaluation in a different setting? Proven evaluation methodologies must be employed in a legitimate evaluation and resources need to be used judiciously. It is advised that HES utilize promising and evidence-based practices to be most impactful. The **propriety standards** are about ensuring that the evaluation is completed ethically, with a focus on equity and fairness. This includes considering what is legal, right, and just in evaluations. For example, was the evaluation carried out with minimal biases? Were multiple methods and strategies used to ensure a complete analysis was conducted? Any limitations are included in this standard. This might include a statement in the final evaluation about how participants were recruited or if a geographic area was not included because it was too far from the program site. This may have actually impacted the program greatly and if replicated without these limitations, then the program results may vary greatly. Finally, **accuracy standards** are focused on the objectivity and truthfulness of the findings. Were the appropriate people included in planning, implementing, and writing the evaluation report? Is the evaluation in a format to serve its intended purpose? Does the report objectively share findings, even if they are unfavorable? Does the report offer unbiased insights about the implementation of the intervention? This is another example when best practices will play an important role in helping HES in developing the format and deciding what content to include.

Activity 4.5: Practice Your Skills

Think about a health education or health promotion program you have either planned on campus or participated in as a student or community member. Answer these questions reflecting on your experience:

1. What was the goal of the program?
2. What type of evaluation could have been completed of the program?
3. What data was gathered to inform an evaluation?
4. Could additional data have been collected? If so, what data?
5. What would you expect in a final report of the program? Would you say it was a success? What could have been improved?

Evaluation Report Writing and Dissemination

The final step in conducting an evaluation is to write the report and share its findings. The final report can take many different forms, anything from a brief one-pager to a four-page research brief, to a journal article, or a multipage report. Considering who will be reading the report, the purpose of the report, and how the report will be used will inform the length, type, content, and format of the final evaluation report.

CDC (2018) recommends that an evaluation report contain seven components, including an executive summary, a background and purpose, a section describing the evaluation methods, the results of the evaluation, a discussion of the results, an overall conclusion with recommendations, and an appendix with examples. The executive summary is generally one to two pages and gives an overall summary of the intervention and contents of the report. It is similar to an abstract in that it highlights key components of the methods and results and shares significant outcomes and findings. The background and purpose section details the need and scope of the intervention. It describes the target population, summarizes needs assessment findings, and lists major goals and objectives. The basis for selecting the given intervention can be discussed and expected benefits can be listed. The evaluation methods section should provide the delineated details of the evaluation plan. This may include the research questions; how, when, and what data is to be collected; who will collect the data and any additional information that would be needed in the event other researchers wanted to replicate your work. If barriers were encountered during the evaluation process, these would be discussed in this section. In the results section of the report, findings are to be listed and described without discussion and analysis. Here, it is helpful to use graphics to illustrate results. Tables, charts, and other tools can provide useful information that the reader can easily understand. In the section that includes the discussion of the results, HES can describe their interpretation of what was found. This can be especially useful if findings varied from what the goals and objectives were initially designed to accomplish. If any data analysis was conducted, the findings can be described and discussed here. While the section with conclusions and recommendations should not introduce any new topics, it is appropriate to restate what was found as well as suggest recommendations about program quality and effectiveness based on lessons learned. Readers of the report, including agency staff, local coalitions, elected officials, members of the target audience, and funders, will want to know if the program is worthy of continued support and effort. Finally, appendices should be included to share items used in the planning, implementation, and evaluation phases of the intervention. Examples can include project maps, data collection tools, work plans, timelines, logic models, and related project materials that were developed specifically for the target population.

Eight Areas of Responsibility for CHES® and MCHES®

Conducting needs assessments and coordinating efforts in developing interventions aligns with the following Areas of Responsibility for CHES® and MCHES®:

Area IV: Evaluation and Research

This Area includes five competencies and 37 sub-competencies for evaluating health promotion interventions and conducting related research (National Commission for Health and Education Credentialing, Inc. [NCHEC], 2020). These include designing evaluation and research plans, managing the collection, analysis, interpretation, and reporting of data and findings (NCHEC, 2020).

To learn more about the Areas of Responsibility, please visit: https://www.nchec.org.

Once an evaluation report has been written, it needs to be disseminated so that others can learn. Avenues for this include local national media; local, state, and national conferences; peer-reviewed journals; and other similar publications. Presenting and sharing intervention impacts and outcomes is considered appropriate and expected professional behavior of HES.

Activity 4.6: Discussion

Access the listing of five reports for the 2013–2018 Fairfax County Community Health Improvement Plan (CHIP) Evaluation at: https://tinyurl.com/4kj2zsns. At the bottom of the webpage, a link is provided for each of the five yearly reports. Please select the *Year 5* report and review it.

After reviewing the evaluation report, please share your responses to the following questions about the information provided:

1. Who is the audience for the final evaluation report of the CHIP?
2. What do you think about the format of the report?
3. What data and outcomes make the report most meaningful?
4. What is missing from this report? What would make the report more useful?

Evaluation of Best Practices and Strategies for Success

While evaluation needs and tools have changed over time, the American Evaluation Association (AEA) has identified a set of broad best practice concepts that can be applied to a wide range of evaluation settings. The practices the AEA promote,

> ...provide a starting point, framework, and set of perspectives to guide evaluators through the often complex and changing environment encountered in the evaluation of public programs. The following practices help ensure that evaluations provide useful and reliable information to program managers, policy makers, and stakeholders...
>
> *(American Evaluation Association [AEA], n.d., para. 4)*

The AEA recommends using culturally competent practices throughout the process, conducting an initial consultation, building-in multiple opportunities for evaluation in a program, having multiple methods of data collection, and developing multiple versions of evaluation findings for interested parties (AEA, n.d.). It is important to be self-aware, sensitive and to recognize and honor norms and values of those who are different from ourselves, such as differences in race, ethnicity, gender, religion, or socioeconomic level. To ensure evaluations capture the perspectives of and offer insight into impacts of the intervention, it is necessary to choose culturally and linguistically appropriate (CLAS) evaluation methods and strategies. One tool to use when working on culturally competent materials is the National CLAS Standards, developed by the U.S. Department of Health and Human Services and Office of Minority Health (n.d.-a). These standards are intended to improve health equity and quality while helping to eliminate disparities by providing a framework for professionals in the healthcare field (U.S. Department of Health and Human Services and Office of Minority Health, n.d.-a). Adding these standards into the program (or intervention) and evaluation design are intentional steps to support these aims.

Begin with the end of the program in mind when developing an evaluation plan. It is important early in the process to meet with community members, program champions, and other invested partners to make sure everyone is in agreement with regard to the who, what, when, where, and how the evaluation activities will occur. When possible, build evaluation components into the intervention itself to ensure ongoing feedback is collected and utilized. For example, it might be helpful to list several process objectives during

> **SIDEBAR: DID YOU KNOW?**
>
> The **National Standards for Culturally and Linguistically Appropriate Services** (CLAS) were developed to increase health equity, increase access to quality health care, and help eliminate healthcare disparities by providing a set of standards for healthcare professionals and agencies to follow. The standards are designed to "...provide effective, equitable, understandable, and respectful quality care and services that are responsive to diverse cultural health beliefs and practices, preferred languages, health literacy, and other communication needs" (U.S. Department of Health and Human Services and Office of Minority Health, n.d.-b, para. 2).
>
> To review the standards, please visit: https://thinkculturalhealth.hhs.gov/assets/pdfs/EnhancedNationalCLASStandards.pdf.

the planning process so that program staff keep these in mind. This will allow for evaluation efforts to include everything that happens before, during, and after the intervention. The use of multiple evaluation methods will help to strengthen the findings. For example, if one method did not yield sufficient data, another method can make up the shortfall or provide additional insight into the barriers, successes, and lessons learned. Invested partners and project staff can also assist with making sure evaluation methods being used are culturally appropriate, suitable for the health topic, reach the target population, and stay within the evaluation timeframe. Creating different versions of the evaluation findings that will meet the needs of diverse interested parties on the outcomes of the program. For example, one partner might want a one-page summary infographic with engagement data and recommended next steps while another might want a 10-page written report with multiple graphic images highlighting the impact on specific members of the target population.

Concept in Action 4.1

Background: *Aisha* (she/her) has a Master's in Public Health with a focus on community health education. She is also a CHES. She supervises a team of four health educators and manages a budget of $500,000 per year for a large company. She has been in the role for three years and came into the role with four years of experience at a prior worksite. In her previous role, she started as a health educator and was ultimately promoted into a manager position. Aisha was hired to her current role to develop a wellness program. She leads a wellness workgroup at the corporation and has led the company to win a national award recognizing their work developing effective worksite wellness programs. She is highly respected at the company and among her team for her ability to collaborate with others. There was a recent outbreak of the flu that has caused a number of staff to miss work. Aisha reports directly to the CEO.

Aisha recently created a three-pronged flu prevention campaign and is in the process of evaluating the program. In previous years, her CEO noted that staff absenteeism rates were much higher than national averages for the months of November through March. Employees cited that flu was the main reason for taking sick days during those months. The program Aisha implemented included hand-washing messaging in all restrooms, posters, and a video about sneezing and coughing into elbows and offering flu shots to employees. She invited the local hospital to come to the worksite and they held three flu shot mini-clinics in September, October, and November. The company paid for the flu shots. She held hand-washing demonstrations and showed videos of people coughing and sneezing safely in staff meetings. Aisha needs to now figure out how to evaluate the effectiveness of her campaign. Her boss wants to know if it makes sense to repeat the same activities next year or make changes. Working with the human resources office, Aisha has several tools and data sources she can utilize for this purpose.

Aisha has many questions at this stage. These include:

1. What type of data have I collected? What does the data tell me?
2. What data is missing? What data can I still collect?
3. What worked well? What needs improvement for next year?

4.   What are some health indicators I can examine over the entire year?
5.   Who are my partners and interested parties? Who wants the results of this program?
6.   What should I include in my final evaluation report? Why should that be included?

Aisha's three-pronged flu prevention campaign kicked off in September and finished in December. The CEO now wants to know if she should budget for the intervention again next year. The costs were minimal, with the cost of the flu shots being the largest budget item. Since absenteeism due to flu during the months of November through March was the initial reason for the intervention, that same data will now be collected every year. Aisha can compare the absenteeism rate due to flu each year to that of all prior years. Other data she might capture includes self-reported hand washing, knowledge and behavior about cough and sneeze etiquette, and employee family member flu rates. She can create a one to two page summary of this data and make it available to the CEO as well as all employees. While the CEO might be most interested in reducing absenteeism, he or she is also likely to care about the overall health of the employees and their use of health insurance during flu season. This can impact the company's health insurance premiums. Aisha also learned during this process that an effective evaluation plan is one that is developed *before* a program is implemented.

Summary

- A comprehensive evaluation plan is an important component of a health education or health promotion program. HES must be able to show the effectiveness and benefits for resources spent. Various community partners and interested parties will want to know what worked and what didn't. An evaluation plan can help identify valuable information to justify future funding for programs that work.
- Formative, process, impact, outcome, and summative evaluations are all types of evaluations that HES can use to assess programs. HES play a key role in identifying which of these will be most helpful in the intervention evaluation process. In some cases, each evaluation type will be utilized to create a robust review of the intervention and determine if and how the program objectives were met. This comprehensive review may help to inform the quality and effectiveness of the current project as well as long-term sustainability and scalability.
- Sharing the evaluation report with invested partners is a key component of the evaluation process. Channels to distribute the results include reports, presentations, publications, and the use of various social media platforms. Public health professionals rely on the sharing of lessons learned to allow continued justification to inform how we work together to improve population health.
- Some strategies to ensure effective program evaluation HES should use culturally competent practices, conduct an initial consultation, build multiple opportunities for evaluation into a program, have multiple methods of data collection, and develop multiple versions of evaluation findings for interested parties.

Web Resources
■ **American Evaluation Association**
  https://www.eval.org/About/What-is-Evaluation
  This professional association website provides useful information about the different types of evaluations and how to find a qualified external evaluator.
■ **CDC Office of Policy, Performance, and Evaluation**
  https://www.cdc.gov/evaluation/
  This CDC website details methods for effective and efficient program evaluations.
■ **The Community Toolbox – Chapter 37**
  https://ctb.ku.edu/en/table-of-contents/evaluate/evaluate-community-interventions
  This chapter in the Community Toolbox provides an overview of program evaluation and resources, such as stories from the field and toolkits.
■ **The Community Toolbox – Chapter 38**
  https://ctb.ku.edu/en/table-of-contents/evaluate/evaluate-community-initiatives
  This chapter in the Community Toolbox offers examples of methods that can be used to evaluate community initiatives and programs and resources, such as stories from the field and toolkits.
■ **Rural Health Information Hub – Module 4**
  https://www.ruralhealthinfo.org/toolkits/rural-toolkit/4/program-evaluation
  This module of the Rural Community Health Toolkit provides information on the importance, design, measures, and challenges of successful program evaluations.

References

American Evaluation Association. (n.d.). *Practices and Methodology.* https://www.eval.org/Policy-Advocacy/Evaluation-Policy-Initiative/Practices-and-Methodology

Centers for Disease Control and Prevention. (1999). Framework for program evaluation in public health. *MMWR*; 48(No. RR-11). https://www.cdc.gov/mmwr/PDF/rr/rr4811.pdf

Centers for Disease Control and Prevention. (2017). *A Framework for Program Evaluation.* https://www.cdc.gov/evaluation/framework/index.htm

Centers for Disease Control and Prevention. (2018). *Evaluation Briefs: Preparing an Evaluation Report.* https://www.cdc.gov/mmwr/PDF/rr/rr4811.pdf

Centers for Disease Control and Prevention. (2021). *Flu Vaccination Coverage, United States, 2020–21 Influenza Season.* https://www.cdc.gov/flu/fluvaxview/coverage-2021estimates.htm

Joint Committee on Standards for Educational Evaluation. (2023). *Program Evaluation Standards.* https://jcsee.org/program/

National Commission for Health and Education Credentialing, Inc. (2020). *Areas of Responsibility, Competencies and Sub-competencies for Health Education Specialist Practice Analysis II 2020 (HESPA II 2020).* https://assets.speakcdn.com/assets/2251/hespa_competencies_and_sub-competencies_052020.pdf

U.S. Department of Health and Human Services & Office of Minority Health. (n.d.-a). *About Us.* https://thinkculturalhealth.hhs.gov/about

U.S. Department of Health and Human Services & Office of Minority Health. (n.d.-b). *National Standards for Culturally and Linguistically Appropriate Services (CLAS) in Health and Health Care.* https://thinkculturalhealth.hhs.gov/assets/pdfs/EnhancedNationalCLASStandards.pdf

Yarbrough, D.B., Shula, L.M., Hopson, R.K., & Caruthers, F.A. (2010). *The Program Evaluation Standards: A Guide for Evaluators and Evaluation Users* (3rd ed.). Corwin Press.

CHAPTER 5

Planning and Implementing Interventions and Programs: Engaging Process for Impact

Learning Objectives

After reading this chapter, learners will be able to:

- Describe the importance of planning for health education and promotion interventions and programs
- Determine best practices for engaging community members and interested parties
- Apply planning tools to the development of health education and promotion interventions and programs
- Recommend strategies to prioritize health equity in program implementation
- Describe individual, organizational, and societal benefits and barriers in implementing health education and promotion interventions and programs

Keywords

- Best Practices
- Budget
- Coalition
- Community Engagement
- Evaluation Phase
- Evidence-Based Recommendations
- Health Impact Pyramid
- Impact Objective
- Implementation Phase
- Outcome Objective
- Planning Committee
- Planning Phase
- Pre-planning Phase
- Process Objective
- Mission Statement
- Steering Committee
- Target Population
- Task Force
- The Community Guide
- Timeline
- Vision Statement
- Work Plan

DOI: 10.4324/9781003504320-5

Self-Reflection Questions

Think about an event that you planned or helped to plan, such as a party. Consider these questions about that experience:

1. Who did you ask to help you with the planning?
2. What were some of the steps you completed?
3. Did the event go as planned? Why or why not?
4. Would you do anything differently next time? If so, why and how?

The delivery of health education and health promotion programs does not happen by chance. Health education includes "...any combination of learning experiences designed to help individuals and communities improve their health by increasing knowledge, influencing motivation and improving health literacy" (World Health Organization [WHO], 2021, p. 18, para. 5). Whereas "...health promotion is the process of enabling people to increase control over, and to improve their health" (WHO, 2021, p. 4, para. 1). Important terms used in these definitions include *combination of learning experiences*, *designed to improve health*, and *process of enabling people*. In order to successfully deliver health education and promotion programs, each of these important components must be considered during the planning process. In addition, decisions about health topics to address, settings, and available resources must be considered during the **planning phase**. Just as a recipe is followed in cooking, a planning model is crucial to the successful implementation of health education and health promotion interventions or programs. This chapter examines using planning tools to engage interested parties and develop sound, effective interventions, and programs.

Terminology in This Chapter

This chapter will focus on planning and implementing health education interventions and programs and health promotion interventions and programs. Sometimes a program may include an intervention, with even a control and test group. Examples of interventions and programs can include small- and large-scale events, training, workshops, and lessons. Rather than specifying the details of an intervention or program to explore the process of planning and implementation, both will be included. For simplicity, the phrases *health education and promotion interventions and programs* and *interventions and programs* will be used to indicate both.

The Importance of Needs Assessments

Before the planning of health education and promotion interventions and programs begins, a needs assessment is completed to identify the health needs and gaps in the community. A Community Health Needs Assessment (CHA) is a formalized and structured process to determine these needs and gaps and this information provides the foundation for the planning and implementation of health education and promotion interventions and programs. CHAs can provide valuable insight, such as:

- What are the top two or three health concerns in the community?
- Who is impacted by these health concerns?
- What is the change we want to see in our community?
- What resources will we need to accomplish our goals?
- How will we know if we were successful?

Answers to these and other questions guide the rest of the planning process and will be included in a Community Health Improvement Plan (CHIP). A CHIP is a detailed plan with identified goals, objectives, and action steps for achieving health outcomes by meeting the needs and addressing the gaps identified in the CHA. A CHIP is usually the end product of a needs assessment process and is referred to throughout the planning process and in evaluation efforts.

Needs Assessments

It may be helpful to review information in Chapter 3 on needs assessments. Chapter 3 provided a few examples of planning models, with the focus on the assessment portion of the model. These models are also used in planning and implementing health education and promotion programs.

Steps in Planning

Assessment is an important part of the planning process because it identifies what the community needs and may include some suggestions and thoughts on how to address them. A CHA may identify multiple needs, some of which may already be included in interventions in the community and others may be incredibly complex to address. To address all of these needs thoughtful planning is required. However, program planning does not happen in a silo. It takes an intentional and collaborative approach.

Although planning models frequently describe the same basic tasks, they may use different names for the phases or steps to be completed. There are five standard steps in program planning (as indicated in Table 5.1). These include pre-planning and needs assessment; developing goals, objectives, and action items; choosing and/or developing interventions; implementing interventions; and evaluating outcomes.

Initial steps include completing the needs assessment in the pre-planning phase. This might involve forming a **planning committee**. This committee may review the results of the needs assessment, conduct a resources and capacity inventory, and propose an intervention or program timeline. Based on the initial findings in the CHA, the next steps include determining desired goals, objectives, and outcomes. This is part of the planning phase. Next, examples of existing programs and recommendations for intervention programs are researched to identify the most appropriate and effective options. Once an intervention or program is chosen or developed, it is implemented in the implementation phase. Although determining evaluation plans and strategies for collecting data are part of the planning process and occur through the intervention and program, the final steps in a planning process incorporate completing a comprehensive evaluation.

Table 5.1 Steps in Planning

Phase	Step	Description
Preplanning	Needs assessment	Form planning group, steering committee; review results of needs assessment(s) including data collected; review resources/capacity; determine intervention timeline
Planning	Developing goals, objectives, and action items	Determine desired outcomes of the intervention or program; assign roles for remaining tasks
	Choosing and/or developing interventions or programs	Research current best practices and evidence-based interventions or programs; conduct a literature review; consult experts in the field
Implementation	Implementing interventions or programs	Deliver chosen intervention(s) or programs as planned and designed; monitor for fidelity; begin formative; and process evaluation
Evaluation	Evaluating outcomes	Conduct process, impact, and outcome evaluation; report findings; determine next steps for continued implementation based on lessons learned

Community Engagement

Community engagement can be defined as "...the process of working collaboratively with and through groups of people affiliated by geographic proximity, special interest, or similar situations to address issues affecting the well-being of those people" (Centers for Disease Control and Prevention [CDC], 1997, p. 9). There are several ways to invite and engage partners and interested parties from the community to the planning process. The terms stakeholders, partners, committee members, interested parties, and community members are used somewhat interchangeably. These terms mainly describe the people who are interested in and engaged in the planning and implementation phases. They are the people invested in the success of the intervention or program. The number and type of interested partners who will participate in planning efforts will vary depending on the size and scope of the community and resources available. At the very least, people invested and interested in addressing specific health topics and those from the community who have been impacted will most likely want to be involved. It is the job of a HES to identify and recruit these partners.

In some cases, members of the planning committee will be paid staff from various businesses and organizations. This might include local hospitals, businesses, nonprofits, schools, government agencies, and institutions of higher education. These partners bring vast and diverse experience, knowledge, and skills to the planning process. Other committee members might be community volunteers who represent themselves as they live, work, pray, or play in the community. Other volunteers from the community may include representatives from local homeowners' associations, civic groups, or other vested parties. These volunteer contributors also bring rich and intimate knowledge of the **target population**. The target population is the subgroup of your community you will hope to reach with your intervention. For example, if you are working on a project to reduce youth vaping, the target population might be middle and high school students. Within the target population, there may be gatekeepers, or people with significant influence. This might include an elected official, faith-based leader, or head of a student government group. The term champions is often used to describe these individuals because they often represent the target population and can provide assistance in gaining access and leading efforts to engage other partners formally and informally.

Additional Planning Groups

Once the planning committee has laid the foundation for the work ahead, additional groups are often formed to assist in the planning and implementation of interventions and programs. This is common because of the sheer volume of work that has been identified and in order to accomplish the goals, multiple partners are needed. The process of establishing these groups can occur over the multiple steps involved in planning and implementing a CHIP. Completing a CHA can take two to three years and implementing a CHIP can take up to five more, depending on what the planning group decides. There may be times when the members of these additional groups overlap with each other. For example, they can include members of the planning committee. However, each planning group has its own purpose and responsibilities. Three additional types of planning groups include steering committees, coalitions, and a task force.

A **steering committee** is a group of invested community partners who are tasked with giving oversight and guidance to a specific project or intervention. Specific membership is determined by the size and scope of the intervention. For example, if the intervention is about diabetes then inviting someone from the local chapter of the American Diabetes Association would be appropriate. Steering committee members might assist in the planning, development, implementation, and evaluation of the intervention. Examples of steering committee member duties include attending meetings, offering ideas and technical or subject matter expertise, and helping to identify and secure needed human and financial resources. When identifying and selecting steering committee members, project staff seek individuals who have a vested interest and expertise in the health topic or may be a part of the target population and considered to be gatekeepers, or leaders within the community that can connect and introduce others to the efforts of the community and project staff. A steering committee may also include paid staff from a variety of businesses and organizations, government entities, community volunteers, and others directly affected by the health topic. A steering committee will continue to meet regularly throughout the lifecycle of the intervention.

SIDEBAR: DID YOU KNOW?

Since 2010, the Partnership for a Healthier Fairfax (PFHF) has been working to assess health needs and implement interventions and programs designed to improve health outcomes (The Official Site of Fairfax County [FFX Co], n.d.). It is a multisector coalition of individuals, organizations, and businesses led by a Steering Committee that works together to address the health needs of its diverse communities through the implementation of a wide variety of community-owned health improvement activities identified in the CHIP (FFX Co, n.d.).

The first CHIP, from 2013 to 2018, included 11 goals and 31 objectives across seven priority health issues (FFX Co, n.d.). By early 2019, over 90% of the key actions were either completed or in progress (FFX Co, n.d.). Successful outcomes included developing a bicycle master plan, establishing tobacco-free play zones, encouraging community gardens and mobile food markets, establishing the Trauma-Informed Community Network, and the development of the Community Health Dashboard. The second CHIP spans across the period of 2019–2023 and addresses community-identified and prioritized health issues. It was developed based on the results of a CHA and subsequent assessments. This plan includes 8 goals and 20 objectives across three priority health issues (FFX Co, n.d.).

The PFHF is an impressive example of how a community can come together to plan and implement health promotion activities that are designed with input from the community. From the initial health needs assessment to the development of a comprehensive CHIP, continued and sustained efforts from multiple invested partners are key.

To learn more about the PFHF, please visit: https://www.fairfaxcounty.gov/live healthy/partnership.

A **coalition** is a group of people who come together to work on or solve a specific problem. Community health coalitions can be successful at improving health outcomes at the local, regional, state, and even national levels (Butterfoss, 2007). Because coalitions bring together a varied group of partners, the health issue can be addressed from multiple angles. Coalitions are successful if they are able to efficiently mobilize members to work together toward a shared and common goal. While similar to steering committees, coalitions usually have a more specific task or tasks that help to move an intervention forward. For example, a steering committee might form a coalition to work on one goal or objective that is part of a larger effort, such as a CHIP. If tobacco control was identified in a CHA as a health concern and the subsequent CHIP has objectives related to tobacco control, a Tobacco Control Coalition may be created to work toward meeting the tobacco-related action items. Creating a coalition may also help to avoid expensive and time-consuming duplication of efforts. For example, a HES might learn that there is already a group of people working on a health issue of interest. Instead of creating a new coalition, the HES can contact the already-existing group and offer to join forces. This can strengthen and improve efforts moving forward. A coalition may meet long term or until its specific goals or objectives are met. Similar to a coalition, a **task force** is a group of people who have been charged with working on a specific problem or issue. A task force may only meet a few times or they may form a longer lasting group. Regardless of what a planning group is called, the tasks and responsibilities are imperative to the overall success of the intervention.

> **Eight Areas of Responsibility for CHES® and MCHES®**
>
> Conducting needs assessments and coordinating efforts in developing interventions align with the following Areas of Responsibility for CHES® and MCHES®.
>
> **Area III: Implementation**
>
> This Area includes three competencies and 16 sub-competencies for implementing health promotion interventions in the community (National Commission for Health and Education Credentialing, Inc. [NCHEC], 2020). This includes coordinating the delivery of interventions, implementing interventions, and the subsequent monitoring of interventions (NCHEC, 2020).
>
> To learn more about the Areas of Responsibility, please visit: https://www.nchec.org.

Planning and Implementation Tools

Regardless of the type of intervention or program that may be replicated or developed while implementing the CHIP, there are planning tools that can help provide clarity, track activities, and ultimately measure success. Some of these are integrated into the planning models, sometimes funders require the use of a specific tool that they have developed and expect feedback on the tools during the implementation stage, and some planning tools are just helpful to the process because they may help to organize the group's actions. These include mission and vision statements, goals and objectives, timeline, and work plan.

Mission and vision statements are two tools that are typically used together to help planning committees and each of the planning groups to guide their work. Each of these groups may want to develop these for their specific tasks and responsibilities to ensure they remain focused on their specific task over a long period of time. These tools can also be used by larger bodies, such as organizations and employers.

A **mission statement** defines the organization or group, states the objectives of the organization or group, and details how the objectives will be reached. For example, the mission statement may be to improve the health of moms and babies through community outreach, education, and resources designed to facilitate prenatal and postpartum care (as indicated in Table 5.2).

Table 5.2 Sample Mission and Vision Statements

Statement Type	Sample Language
Mission statement	The mission of the Healthy Moms and Babies initiative is to improve the health of moms and babies through community outreach, education, and resources designed to facilitate prenatal and postpartum care.
Vision Statement	A community where all pregnant people, postpartum people, infants, and children have the opportunity to thrive and live their healthiest lives.

A **vision statement** details where the group hopes to go. For example, (as indicated in Table 5.2) the vision can be a community where all pregnant people, postpartum people, infants, and children have the opportunity to thrive and live their healthiest lives. The mission and vision statements help to clarify why the group has formed and what they hope to accomplish in the near to mid future. Mission and vision statements are most impactful when they are created, agreed upon, and voted on by invested partners in the planning phase.

Activity 5.1: Practice Your Skills

Go to the homepage of your college or university website and search for the mission and vision statements. Review these and then consider your responses to the following questions:

a. How are the values stated in the mission and vision represented in your interactions with your school?
b. How are the values represented in how your school promotes itself?

Repeat this activity for another organization in your community, such as a faith-based organization or a social service agency. Share and discuss your findings.

After reviewing the results of the CHA, many planning committees will identify a goal. The goal is an overarching statement of what the group hopes to accomplish. Goals provide a general idea and direction of the purpose of the intervention (as indicated in Table 5.3). For example, the goal can be to increase physical activity. A program, referred to as an initiative in this example, can have more than one goal. For example, the goals of a Healthy Moms and Babies initiative might be to reduce infant mortality and improve maternal health. Goal statements are visionary in some ways because these are not things that can typically be achieved in a matter of a few years. They are aspirational and inspirational and yet they guide the work to be done.

Once a goal statement or statements have been agreed upon (usually in the pre-planning phase), objectives and action steps to work toward the goal(s) need to be developed. These action steps are often referred to as objectives. Each goal statement can have one or more objectives and key action items. Interventions and programs may be complex and address more than one goal. Objectives detail the very specific steps that will need to occur to work toward the goal. Objectives are most useful when they are realistic and designed to be achieved during the implementation phase. There are three main types of objectives: process, impact, and outcome.

Process objectives describe how to complete the intended activities of the intervention or program. For example, for the Bridgeport Rides! example, a process objective

Table 5.3 Sample Goal Statements

Sample Goal Statements
The goal of the Bridgeport Rides! Program is to increase physical activity.
The two goals of the Healthy Moms and Babies initiative are to reduce infant mortality and improve maternal health.

might be how many worksites are going to be contacted and invited to join the coalition. For the Healthy Moms and Babies example, a process objective might include the number of pregnant women the intervention plans to reach in the first year or how many prenatal clinics will be contacted and invited to serve as partner referral sites by the end of the second year. Process objectives identify specific metrics to achieve while working toward the goal. **Impact objectives** describe what changes are expected in behavior, knowledge, attitude, or environment. In the Bridgeport Rides! example, an impact objective might be about how many adults will report that they bike to work after the intervention as compared to before the intervention, indicating a change in their behavior. For the Healthy Moms and Babies example, an impact objective might be how many pregnant people demonstrate that they know the importance of prenatal care after the intervention and can list at least five benefits of breastfeeding, indicating a change in knowledge at the conclusion of the educational sessions. Finally, **outcome objectives** are developed to measure a longer-term change in a health indicator or outcome. For example, a reduction in obesity rates, a decrease in the number of low birth weight babies, or a decrease in the infant mortality rate in a given state. Outcome objectives are typically measured after the intervention or program ends because these kinds of changes in health outcomes take time to show a significant change. Many data systems update these kinds of data every few years.

In order to be impactful, useful, and measurable, each of these types of objectives needs to be SMART: Specific, Measurable, Attainable, Realistic, and Time-bound (Doran, 1981). SMART objectives (as indicated in Table 5.4) answer the questions, who will do what, by how much, and by when.

Questions to consider for developing *Specific* objectives include:

- What is the exact activity or change that is desired?
- What is the population that is expected to meet the objective? 100% of high school students? 80% of program participants?
- What do they need to do? Perhaps the participants will be able to report biking to work at least two days per week?

Table 5.4 SMART Objectives

Type of Objective	Sample Language
Process	By December 31, project staff will contact at least 15 OB/GYN offices.
	By March 31, at least 50 pregnant moms will be enrolled in the Healthy Moms and Babies intervention.
Impact	By December 31, 90% of the enrolled moms will report taking prenatal vitamins daily.
	By March 31, 75% of enrolled moms will be able to list five benefits of receiving regular prenatal care.
Outcome	By the end of 2025, there will be a 15% reduction in low birth weight babies.
	By the end of 2025, there will be a 10% reduction in the infant mortality rate in the state.

Questions to consider for developing *Measurable* objectives include:

- How will the objective be measured? By attendance? Test score? Weight loss?
- Will there be a pre- and a post-test?
- Is an increase or decrease expected? If so, by how much? Is a 10% increase expected?

Questions to consider for developing *Attainable* objectives include:

- Can the desired change happen in the time allotted?
- Is it an appropriate expectation given the parameters of the intervention?

Questions to consider for developing *Realistic* objectives include:

- Will the population be able to meet the objective?
- Are there external forces that will prohibit the success of the intervention?

Questions to consider for developing *Time-bound* objectives include:

- When is the activity or change due? By the end of the year? By the end of the program? Within three months of beginning the program?

Developing SMART objectives is an important step in the planning phase because objectives serve as the foundation for designing a successful intervention.

A **timeline** is another important tool in planning and implementing interventions and programs. A timeline is useful because it can lay out each component and aspect of what is needed to carry out the key steps, monitor the overall process, identify staffing needs and roles, identify and include training opportunities, consider when to acquire materials and supplies, and review the dates of the delivery and evaluation of the intervention or program. A timeline includes details about when each activity is scheduled to occur. Because things do not always go as planned, a timeline can be adjusted throughout the implementation process. Since the timeline has each activity included, it can help to make sure steps aren't missed if one or more of the activities take longer than originally expected. Hiring staff is a great example of this. While it may seem relatively simple to post a job description and hire someone, in reality, it can take one to three months. If every step is contingent on when someone is hired, then the remaining steps can be adjusted to accommodate a lengthy search process.

Another useful tool that can be used to organize activities and the time allotted for each into one concise document is a **work plan**. A well-written work plan, as indicated in Figure 5.1, includes the program goals, measurable objectives, action items or key tasks, the responsible party or lead person for each task, and the time allotted for each task. Most external funders require a work plan be submitted with a grant application as a proposed plan for how the program is expected to be executed. Work plans can encompass one or more years of the funding cycle and may be necessary when there are complex objectives to meet.

Finally, a **budget** is a necessary tool for HES to use as part of successfully managing the implementation phase of an intervention or program. Proposed budgets are always

Goal 1: Significantly increase the number of adults participating in regular physical activity.
SMART Objectives:
1. Increase the number of worksites who offer fitness classes on-site by 20.
2. Increase the number of fitness classes offered by the Parks and Recreation department by five per month.

Objective	Key Tasks	Lead	1	2	3	4	5	6	7	8	9	10	11	12
			Timeframe in months (12)											
1.1.1	Conduct an environmental scan to see which worksites currently offer on-site fitness classes.	HES	x	x										
1.1.2	Prepare and disseminate a toolkit to assist worksites in how to offer on-site fitness classes.	HES				x	x	x		x	x	x		
1.1.3	Convene a fitness intervention Task Force to survey adults in the community on what new fitness interventions are desired.	HES and Fitness Intervention Task Force	x	x	x									
1.1.4	The Task Force to meet bi-monthly.	Fitness Intervention Task Force		x		x		x		x		x		x
1.2.1	Conduct a review of current adult fitness classes being offered by the Parks and Recreation department.	HES	X	X	X									
1.2.1	Use results of surveys to determine what type and number of new fitness classes will be offered by the Parks and Recreation Dept.	HES and Fitness Intervention Task Force				X	X	X						

Figure 5.1 Sample Work Plan and Timeline

provided to a funder to identify the anticipated expenses and revenue. A detailed budget also provides the project staff and planning groups with a plan of how the grant or other funds will be allocated over the course of the implementation of the intervention or program. Internally funded interventions almost always include a budget as well. Local and state health departments often implement interventions using federal, state, or local funding from foundations or other organizations that are interested in the successful implementation of interventions and programs. Being accountable to all

Table 5.5 Budget Categories

Budget Category	Examples of Items Included
Personnel	Organization staff and independent contractors who are directly involved in the intervention, fringe benefits, and other payroll costs
Travel	Mileage, hotel, meals, and airfare related to training or other required travel
Materials and Supplies	Expendable items such as food, paper, pens, curricula, incentives, giveaways, and promotional materials
Equipment	Durable goods such as computers, printers, cell phones, display tables, and office furniture
Printing and Marketing	Printing of flyers and brochures, internet and social media advertising, and website design
Indirect Costs	Costs that an organization incurs that are not directly related to the implementation, such as part of the salary of a person who works in accounts payable and manages the spending of the funds, internet subscriptions, and electricity
Match	Funds or other resources that are offered in-kind, free of charge, that are considered a gift, such as office space, time for staff to attend coalition meetings, and use of a copier.
Revenue	Projected revenue or earned income from sources such as admission tickets, sale of products, and monetary donations

possible funders and funding sources is critical to the implementation, evaluation, and sustainability of interventions.

Budgets can vary in size and scope, but most will include eight categories, as indicated in Table 5.5. The categories include personnel, travel, materials and supplies, equipment, printing and marketing, indirect costs, match, and revenue.

Personnel costs can include project staff (directors, managers, and front-line staff) and independent contractors (also known as consultants). This category includes fringe benefits and other taxes and required deductions for employees. The travel category includes any project-related expenses, such as mileage, tolls, airfare, lodging, etc. Materials and supplies are generally the items that will be consumed or distributed to participants during the intervention or program. Therefore, these items will be used and will no longer be available after the intervention or program is completed. Equipment is generally considered to be items that will continue to have a life after the intervention ends, such as cookware or a laptop. The printing and marketing category includes any flyers, posters, or postcards that will be needed. One question to ask here is, will the printing be done in-house or will it be sent to a commercial printer? Some agencies have a printer and can handle large print jobs, while others do not. The print job could also involve printing on a banner or on t-shirts. These will need to be done by another business. Indirect costs are those costs that are not directly related to the day-to-day implementation of the intervention; however, they are needed to support the work. For example, a person who works in accounts payable may charge 5% of their time to the project budget as he or she is responsible for paying project staff and invoices. Some budgets include a category called match. This includes a listing of in-kind contributions from partners. An example might be the administrative support that an assistant from another agency offers as their commitment to the project. It can also be a donation of whistles that were left over from another organization's event last year and rather than discarding them they could be used in the implementation of an intervention or program at the local high school. Finally, budgets may include projected revenue, as appropriate. This may not occur because generally the costs to host and implement an intervention or program are all included in a budget that is internally or externally funded. If HES were to collect any funds for participating in an intervention or program, they must follow the fiscal guidelines to ensure the money is accounted for and deposited properly. While not all interventions generate revenue, it is a way to demonstrate how an intervention might sustain itself after initial funding goes away.

Selecting and Developing Interventions

For many HES, selecting an existing intervention or program or developing a new intervention or program is when the exciting work begins. Regardless of which path is taken, there are several factors to be considered for successful implementation. Two of these, the Health Impact Pyramid and the Community Guide, will be discussed next.

The **Health Impact Pyramid (HIP)**, indicated in Figure 5.2, is a framework that can be used to assist in the selection of interventions and programs. The HIP illustrates the kind of impact an intervention or program is likely to have on an individual or a community (Frieden, 2010). The HIP also highlights examples of efforts that can have a positive impact on health equity. CDC explains that "health equity is the state in which everyone has a fair and just opportunity to attain their highest level of health" (2022, para. 1). In order for HES and public health professionals to make a significant impact on the health of a community or population, it is imperative that interventions and

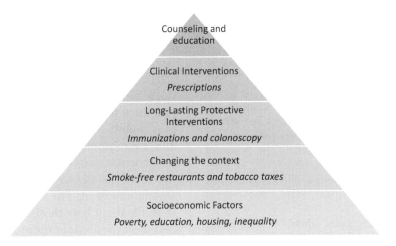

Figure 5.2 The Health Impact Pyramid

Note: Adapted from "A Framework for Public Health Action: The Health Impact Pyramid." by Thomas R. Frieden, 2010, American Journal of Public Health: April 2010, Vol. 100, No. 4, pp. 590–595. https://doi.org/10.2105/AJPH.2009.185652. Retrieved from https://www.ncbi.nlm. nih.gov/pmc/articles/PMC2836340/.

programs are designed to reach diverse groups, including underserved, marginalized, and harder to reach communities. This is an example of working toward health equity.

The Health Impact Pyramid

The base, or foundation, of the HIP is labeled with socioeconomic factors. These can also be referred to as the Social Determinants of Health (SDoH). SDoH are the "… conditions in which people are born, grow, work, live, and age, and the wider set of forces and systems shaping the conditions of daily life" (CDC, 2021, para. 1). These are considered root causes of negative health indicators and outcomes and interventions and programs that positively affect these have the potential to have the greatest impact on health. Income and education levels are highly correlated to health. As income and education levels increase, health improves. This is connected to everything from access to quality health care to improved housing to increased access to healthy foods. In addition, people who are worried about paying their housing and utility bills on a monthly basis may forgo a healthcare visit or fill a prescription. Therefore, interventions that work to improve the SDoH may have greater impacts than those addressing health issues alone.

As each level of the pyramid moves closer to the top, the possibility that the interventions and programs become less impactful at a population level increases. In other words, interventions at the top of the HIP affect small numbers of people while those at the bottom affect large numbers of people. This does not mean that they are not important or less valuable. It simply means that public health professionals can allocate resources based on the goals of a particular intervention, which were developed ideally to address a specific community need. The HIP allows HES to think about how those resources can best meet the needs of the most numbers of people. The *Changing the context* and *Long-lasting protective intervention* levels of the HIP include policy and environmental changes that enable for the healthy or healthier choice to be an

---

SIDEBAR: DID YOU KNOW?

Safe Routes to School is a national health promotion program that strives to make it safe, convenient, and fun for children to walk and bicycle to and from schools. The goal is to get more children walking and bicycling to school, improve kids' safety, and increase health and physical activity (Safe Routes Partnerships [Safe Routes], n.d.).

Children are more sedentary now than at any time in the past. In 1969, nearly 50% of all children in the United States walked or rode bikes to school (Safe Routes, n.d.). Today, that number has plummeted to fewer than 15% (Safe Routes, n.d.). Safe Routes to School programs have been evaluated and proven to be successful at increasing rates of bicycling and walking to school (Safe Routes, n.d.).

Locally, Safe Routes to School staff support advocacy initiatives for strong policies that help make walking and bicycling to school safer. The program includes evaluation, education, encouragement, engineering, enforcement, and equity at the local, state, and federal levels.

To learn more about this national initiative and examples of how it has been successfully implemented in communities across the United States, please visit: https://saferoutespartnership.org/safe-routes-school.

easier choice. Certainly what is considered easier is relative to each person's lived experiences, access to resources, and knowledge. Worksite wellness policies, recommended screenings based on age, and protected bike lanes are all examples of interventions that promote health for everyone. Policy changes are designed to protect all people, regardless of their SDoH. Again, an individual needs to have an employer that offers recommended screenings and the employee needs to feel comfortable getting a screening, but the point is that if implemented well, these strategies have the possibility of having an impact. A classic example is when breakfast cereal companies started adding folic acid (or folate) to cereals. This enrichment of nutrients allowed for females of child-bearing age to reap the benefits of this supplement, which has been proven to help reduce birth defects (March of Dimes, 2020).

The top two levels of the HIP focus more on individual or small group-level interventions. These may include behavioral counseling for weight loss, prescription medication for health conditions, and chronic disease self-management programs. These interventions tend to cost more as they are targeting people who are at a higher risk or may already have a chronic condition. It may require health insurance to be cost-effective and the ability to pay for out-of-pocket expenses. Because these interventions target fewer people, they are considered less impactful on population-level health. As HES look to make significant improvements on health, the HIP can be used as a guide for channeling resources to where they will make the biggest difference. Many communities use multiple strategies across these areas.

The Community Guide

HES have many resources that can help them select the best intervention or program for the health topic and target population. These are known as **best practices** and **evidence-based recommendations** for interventions and programs. Best practices are interventions that are currently being implemented and showing signs of success. Evidence-based recommendations are interventions and programs that have been well-researched and proven to be effective when replicated.

The Community Guide is a free and comprehensive resource that lists evidence-based interventions and programs by topic and population. The information in the Community Guide can be used to research, compare, and ultimately select interventions and programs to improve health and prevent disease in a variety of populations and settings. The Community Guide, based on strict scientific research, can be used to identify and search for health interventions for behavior change, disease prevention, and environmental change; identify areas where more research is needed; and support and supplement decision-making tools, such as HP2030 (Guide to Community Preventive Services [Community Guide], 2023a, para. 1–4).

The Community Preventive Services Task Force (CPSTF), which leads the Community Guide, was established in 1996 by the U.S. Department of Health and Human Services to regularly review current research findings across a wide range of health topics (Community Guide, 2023b). The group is tasked with developing recommendations and guidance on which community-based health promotion and disease prevention intervention approaches work and which do not work (Community Guide, 2023b).

Activity 5.2: Practice Your Skills

The Community Guide is an excellent resource for HES and communities who want to identify evidence-based strategies. Suppose you are a HES recommended strategies for addressing increasing breast cancer rates in your community. You will begin by reviewing the Community Guide at: https://www.thecommunityguide.org.

- Type *asthma* in the search box or select *asthma* from the list of topics.
- Next, locate the *Summary Table* that includes the summary of the Task Force Findings.
- Then, review the interventions and programs that are *recommended*. Review the details of the intervention or program the reasons why they were each found to be effective.
- Next, locate the interventions or programs that have *insufficient evidence*. This means that the efforts did not demonstrate that they could impact health outcomes in a significant way currently. Review each of these interventions and programs to learn why they are not recommended.
- Then, review the available tools to assist with planning interventions and programs on asthma. This includes the one-pagers and a fact sheet on strategies for addressing asthma.
- Select *In Action Stories* to review examples of success stories related to implementing interventions and programs on breast cancer.
- Repeat this process for another health topic of your choosing.

Considerations for Interventions and Programs

There are many things for HES to consider in the planning and implementation of interventions and programs. This includes the level of prevention being addressed, whether a new or existing intervention or program will be implemented, and the type of intervention or program to implement.

Levels of Prevention

Interventions and programs can be categorized into three levels of prevention: primary, secondary, and tertiary (WHO, 2023). It is important to consider these different levels of prevention because HES cannot treat all people the same – everyone is at a different place. Some individuals will want to prevent cancer, some have cancer and want to prevent the toll of stress on their health, and some want to prevent cancer from coming back. Identifying which level to address will shape the intervention or program delivery (Table 5.6).

Primary prevention activities are designed to promote health and prevent disease. These include strategies such as those that increase physical activity, improve diets, increase vaccine uptake, and encourage regular healthcare check-ups. Secondary prevention initiatives include those that identify people at a high risk for disease and provide early diagnosis and treatment to manage and perhaps reverse or cure an illness. Examples include a wide range of cancer screenings, blood tests, and encouragement of early visits to healthcare providers when signs and symptoms are present. The goal of tertiary prevention is to manage disease and illness that has progressed in an effort to allow the person to maintain as high of a quality of life as possible. This might include cardiac or respiratory rehabilitation, surgery, and chronic disease self-management programs.

Table 5.6 Levels of Prevention

Level	Description
Primary	Designed to promote health and prevent disease
Secondary	Designed for people at a high risk for disease to provide early diagnosis, treatment, or cure for an illness
Tertiary	Designed to manage disease and illness that has progressed

Activity 5.3: Discussion
Effective interventions and programs are accessible to diverse groups and address knowledge, attitudes, beliefs, and behaviors at multiple levels. Therefore, an intervention or program that addresses each category of primary, secondary, and tertiary prevention may impact more individuals.

1. Suppose you are a HES working with students. What would be an example of a primary prevention intervention or program that might be appropriate for high school students? College students? Employees in their 40s and 50s?
2. Suppose you are a HES working with older adults living in an assisted living facility. What would be an example of an intervention or program that would meet all three levels of prevention?

Existing and New

Within each level of prevention, there are many types of interventions and programs that can be selected or designed. Selecting an intervention or program is choosing an existing intervention or program already in place in the community that may just need to be revised or enhanced to meet the needs of the community identified in the CHA and CHIP. HES can also choose to duplicate an existing intervention that already exists in another community. There are several benefits for choosing an intervention that already exists including, but not limited to, the time and resources necessary to create a brand new program may not be needed. The existing intervention might have an evaluation component already built into it that can be easily modified. These are all valuable time savers. However, these programs may be expensive to implement or may not be a good fit for the specific community needs being addressed. When creating a new intervention or program, HES must be ready to conduct the research needed to fully develop the intervention or program. It will take time to develop, test, and implement the training and materials needed for a new intervention or program.

Activity 5.4: Practice Your Skills
Regardless of whether a new or existing intervention or program is selected, it needs to be inclusive in design. One tool to assist with this is the National Standards for Culturally and Linguistically Appropriate Services (CLAS) in Health and Health Care located

online at: https://thinkculturalhealth.hhs.gov/assets/pdfs/EnhancedNationalCLASStandards.
pdf. Review the standards and consider how you would implement the standards.

1. As a HES, what would you do to ensure that demographic data is collected and is accurate?
2. As a HES, what practices would you employ to ensure you are developing cultural and linguistic appropriate interventions and programs?

Types of Interventions and Programs

There are five main types of interventions or programs based on the activities involved. These include individual or group education, health communication, environmental, policy, and community engagement.

At the individual or small group education type, school or worksite classes are common. Patients receiving health education upon discharge from a hospital, an individual reading a health brochure, and people attending a falls prevention class are examples. An intervention that includes daily, tailored text messages is another intervention designed for individuals. Some interventions fall under the category of health communication. These include television and print advertisements, pop-up messages on social media, and other communication channels. Environmental interventions target the built environment, or human-made changes that help make healthier choices easier. Examples are healthy vending machines, trails and bike lanes, bike racks, locker rooms at worksites, and parks and playgrounds. Interventions at the policy level can have huge impacts as policies usually cover large groups of people or even total populations. Indoor smoking bans, increased age requirements to buy alcohol and tobacco products and air and water pollution standards are examples. Finally, some interventions are designed to impact at the community level. These might include health coalitions, grassroots campaigns, and other advocacy efforts (Table 5.7).

SIDEBAR: DID YOU KNOW?

The National Action Plan to Improve Health Literacy was released in May 2010 by the U.S. Department of Health and Human Services and was designed to improve health literacy across sectors and communities (2010). The main tenets of the plan are "... that (1) everyone has the right to health information that helps them make informed decisions and (2) health services should be delivered in ways that are understandable and beneficial to health, longevity, and quality of life" (2010, para. 2).

To learn more and review the plan, please visit: https://health.gov/our-work/national-health-initiatives/health-literacy/national-action-plan-improve-health-literacy.

Benefits and Barriers of Implementing Interventions and Programs

The role of HES can vary; however, most HES are hired to plan and implement health education and promotion interventions and programs with the hope of affecting the leading causes of preventable death, such as heart disease, cancer, diabetes, and diseases of the lungs. However, while the work of changing knowledge may seem easy – changing behaviors is hard work. In addition, changing policies and systems can be equally as difficult. It is also very difficult

Table 5.7 Main Types of Health Education and Promotion Interventions and Programs

Type of Intervention or Program	Examples
Individual or group education	▪ Tobacco cessation ▪ School health curricula ▪ Worksite seminars ▪ Diabetes education ▪ Chronic disease self-management
Health communication	▪ National, regional, and local ▪ Social media ▪ TV ▪ Print
Environmental	▪ Bike lanes and racks ▪ Enhanced trails ▪ Water bottle filling stations
Policy	▪ Tax on sugary beverages ▪ Indoor air smoking bans ▪ Gun safety regulations ▪ Clean air and water policies
Community engagement	▪ Grassroots campaigns ▪ Coalitions ▪ Advocacy

to prove that the efforts of a HES contributed to preventing something. How can we know if a specific intervention or program caused more people to get vaccinated? Was it because members of a community were scared about the hospitalization rates? Was it because they heard the vaccine was available at the local pharmacy? Or was it because they had a speaker at their last community meeting who urged them to get vaccinated?

At the individual level, behavior change can be easy to measure. Programs can be tailored to meet the needs and characteristics of individuals. A great example of this is the Text4Baby program sponsored by Wellpass. Pregnant and new parents, their friends, and family members can sign up to receive free text messages in English or Spanish multiple times per week about what to expect during specific points in a pregnancy and post-pregnancy (Text4Baby, 2017). Most cell phone carriers provide the messages with no charge for the data usage, and the messages are created by prenatal experts and tailored to the baby's due date (Text4Baby, 2017). Some topics covered by the text messages include nutrition, signs and symptoms of labor, safe sleep tips, growth and development milestones, breastfeeding tips, and more.

Activity 5.5: Discussion

Go to the website, https://www.text4baby.org, and review the details of the Text4Baby program. Then consider your response to the following questions:

1. How easy is it to sign up for the program?
2. What other health issues can you think of that would align well with a text messaging program? Do these already exist?

3. Do you use a social media platform to improve your health?
4. What are the benefits and barriers of text-based interventions and programs?

While individual-level interventions and programs can be highly successful, some barriers include identifying high-quality examples that are evidence-based. Examples of implemented evidence-based interventions and programs are not always easy to find, especially in more rural areas. Additional barriers may include cost, time, program location, transportation options, and health insurance status. Some program participants may also be hesitant to provide personal information or sign an informed consent document making recruitment challenging.

At the organizational level, schools and workplaces can be effective settings as the target population is already on-site. In schools, while HES might compete for program time with required academic courses, many health-related interventions and programs can be integrated into existing curricula. One example of how to integrate health education into a school system is the Sandy Hook Promise *Start with Hello* curriculum designed for grades K-5 to which "teaches students to be more socially inclusive and connected to each other" and end isolation (2023, para. 2).

Worksites can also hire HES to provide health and wellness programming in the form of lunch and learn presentations and on-demand health education modules. HES may be hired to review their existing vending and meeting foods policies and, as a result, suggest ways to include more health options and connect the leadership to potential new vendors. Finally, worksites can offer health risk assessments at annual health fairs to employees.

Some barriers to providing health education and promotion interventions and programs at worksites include workforce diversity, confidentiality, and privacy. Workplaces are incredibly diverse places when differences in culture, age, and other demographics are considered. This will require intentionality to create inclusive interventions and programs. Depending on the knowledge and skills of HES working on this type of project, it may require additional preparation to understand cultural considerations and the vulnerabilities of various groups. Depending on the workplace, previous interventions and programs may not have had this type of approach and that may feel uncomfortable. Nonetheless, the rewards of engaging in this meaningful approach to health equity are the ethical responsibility of HES. Barriers should not be considered to be impenetrable walls. Other challenges may include employees who may be hesitant to disclose health information to employers for fear of retaliation in the form of higher health insurance premiums or even job loss. Employees may also be suspicious if a worksite brings multiple changes in a short period of time. This might be due to new leadership or a desire to reduce health insurance premiums. Both schools and worksites will have more success if they are fully transparent and forthcoming with information about the purpose and scope of new health-related interventions.

Table 5.8 Social-Ecological Model Levels

Levels of Influence	
Individual	Organization
Family	Policy
Community	

Note: Adapted from "The social ecology of health promotion interventions." by McLeroy, K. R., Steckler, A. and Bibeau, D. (Eds.) (1988). Health Education Quarterly, 15(4):351–377. Retrieved from http://tamhsc.academia.edu/KennethMcLeroy/Papers/81901/An_Ecological_Perspective_on_Health_Promotion_Programs.

At the society level, comprehensive health campaigns can be very successful. Direction can be taken from the social-ecological model of behavior change and interventions can include strategies at multiple levels (individual, family, community, organization, and policy), as indicated in Table 5.8.

Comprehensive tobacco control campaigns are a great example of this concept. Tobacco prevention programs are offered in schools, tobacco cessation tools are offered at worksites, indoor smoking bans are instituted at restaurants and public buildings, mass media campaigns are developed and promoted, sales taxes are increased on tobacco products, and a policy that the age at which people can purchase tobacco products is passed. All of these strategies combined can have and have had significant impacts on decreasing the rate of smoking in the United States (Rhoads, 2012). Collectively, public health and other entities have changed the norms about smoking. It is not the socially accepted behavior that it once was. As the leading preventable cause of death and disease, smoking has been a targeted health behavior for decades.

One important barrier to think about is when we as a society send mixed signals about health behaviors. An example is alcohol consumption. Over 140,000 people die from alcohol-related causes annually in the United States, making alcohol the third-leading preventable cause of death (CDC, 2022). Drinking alcohol is normalized through family gatherings, college parties, sporting events, and other social activities. Television, social media, and print advertising also promote messages about drinking alcohol. These media campaigns can be found everywhere and promote the idea that drinking alcohol is normal and expected in our society. HES must be aware of these types of marketing tactics when designing interventions. It can be challenging to compete with companies that spend billions of dollars promoting behaviors that public health is trying to prevent, or at least minimize.

There are important benefits to health-promoting interventions and programs that can be easy to list. Public health professionals have decades of science and research to support how behavior and lifestyle choices impact health. HES must also keep in mind the barriers faced at all levels of health promotion programming. By using some of that same science and research, HES can overcome these barriers by focusing interventions on data and proven outcomes.

Concept in Action 5.1

Background: José (he/him) manages two community health coalitions and works on several chronic disease prevention interventions in his role at the local health department. He has recently been assigned the additional task of managing the development of the next CHIP. José knows that the well-executed and detailed CHA that was recently completed will make the job of drafting the CHIP a lot easier. He also knows that choosing a planning model that will serve the needs of the community will provide guidance on the process of the CHIP. To engage a diverse group of partners, José will engage members from the two coalitions but will also need to reach out to some new people to form a planning committee. He wants to make sure the planning committee for the CHIP accurately represents his diverse community and that the CHIP represents initiatives that impact health equity.

Fast forward six months…well, José did it! He chose to use the MAPP planning tool that allowed him to expand on his initial needs assessment work. He reached out to members of his current coalitions and several people volunteered to help him with the new CHIP. He also asked each person to think about another person they could invite to become new members of the new coalition. This allowed him to bring some fresh ideas and renewed enthusiasm to the project. The group then developed mission and vision statements and voted on priority issue areas based on activities that focus on ensuring health equity within his community. They are now working on drafting the goals and objectives. Once these are finalized, the newly formed coalition will select appropriate interventions and create a three-year work plan to share with invested partners.

Summary

- Sound, well-thought-out intervention and program planning occur when invested partners come together to solve complex health problems. HES rely on the expertise of these partners to develop and implement interventions that improve population health.

- Steering committees, coalitions, and task forces are examples of some of the additional planning groups that assist in the planning and implementation of interventions and programs and are opportunities for community engagement in the often complex and lengthy process of implementing a CHIP.

- Planning and implementation tools can assist HES in tracking and measuring activities and successes. These include mission and vision statements, goals, objectives, timelines, work plans, and budgets.

- Interventions that address the root causes of health issues and health disparities can positively affect health equity. The Health Impact Pyramid is a framework that can help HES plan interventions that have the greatest impact.

- Just as there are many benefits to implementing interventions and programs, there are some barriers. HES must be aware of potential barriers, such as cost, transportation, privacy issues, and cultural differences, and work to reduce them as much as possible. By doing so, HES can facilitate increased participation in programs designed to improve health outcomes.

Web Resources
- **U.S. Preventive Services Task Force**

  https://www.ahrq.gov/cpi/about/otherwebsites/uspstf/index.html

  This website shares prevention and evidence-based interventions that work to improve the health of all Americans by making recommendations about clinical preventive services such as screenings, counseling services, or preventive medications.
- **Evidence-based Resources**

  https://health.gov/healthypeople/tools-action/browse-evidence-based-resources

  This resource on the Healthy People website lists reviews of health interventions by topic.

References

Butterfoss, F.D. (2007). *Coalitions and Partnerships in Community Health*. John Wiley & Sons.

Centers for Disease Control and Prevention. (1997). *Principles of Community Engagement* (1st ed.). CDC/ATSDR Committee on Community Engagement. Atlanta, GA.

Centers for Disease Control and Prevention. (2021). *Social Determinants of Health*. https://www.cdc.gov/socialdeterminants/index.htm

Centers for Disease Control and Prevention. (2022). *What is Health Equity?* https://www.cdc.gov/healthequity/whatis/index.html

Doran, G.T. (1981). There's a S.M.A.R.T. way to write management's goals and objectives. *Management Review, 70*(11), 35–36.

Guide to Community Preventive Services. (2023a). *About the Community Guide*. https://www.thecommunityguide.org/pages/about-community-guide.html

Guide to Community Preventive Services. (2023b). *About the Community Preventative Services Task Force*. https://www.thecommunityguide.org/pages/about-community-guide.html

Frieden, T.R. (2010). A framework for public health action: The health impact pyramid. *American Journal of Public Health, 100*(4), 590–595. https://doi.org/10.2105/AJPH.2009.185652

March of Dimes. (2020). *Folic Acid*. https://www.marchofdimes.org/find-support/topics/pregnancy/folic-acid

McLeroy, K. R., Steckler, A., & Bibeau, D. (1988). An ecological perspective on health promotion programs. *Health Education Quarterly, 15*(4), 351–377. http://tamhsc.academia.edu/KennethMcLeroy/Papers/81901/An_Ecological_Perspective_on_Health_Promotion_Programs

National Commission for Health and Education Credentialing, Inc. (2020). *Areas of Responsibility, Competencies and Sub-competencies for Health Education Specialist Practice Analysis II 2020 (HESPA II 2020)*. https://assets.speakcdn.com/assets/2251/hespa_competencies_and_sub-competencies_052020.pdf

Rhoads, J.K. (2012). The effect of comprehensive state tobacco control programs on adult cigarette smoking. *Journal of Health Economics, 31*(2), 393–405. https://doi.org/10.1016/j.jhealeco.2012.02.005

Safe Routes Partnerships. (n.d.). *Safe Routes to School*. https://saferoutespartnership.org/safe-routes-school

Sandy Hook Promise. (2023). *Start with Hello*. https://www.sandyhookpromise.org/our-programs/start-with-hello/

Text4Baby. (2017). *Frequently Asked Questions*. https://www.text4baby.org/about/faq

The Official Site of Fairfax County. (n.d.). *Partnership for a Healthier Fairfax*. https://www.fairfaxcounty.gov/livehealthy/partnership

U.S. Department of Health and Human Services. (2010). *National Action Plan to Improve Health Literacy.* Washington, DC. https://health.gov/our-work/national-health-initiatives/health-literacy/national-action-plan-improve-health-literacy

World Health Organization. (2021). *Health Promotion Glossary of Terms.* https://iris.who.int/bitstream/handle/10665/350161/9789240038349-eng.pdf?seqence=1

World Health Organization. (2023). *About Us.* https://www.emro.who.int/about-who/public-health-functions/health-promotion-disease-prevention.html

CHAPTER 6

Advocating: Working Toward Change

Learning Objectives

After reading this chapter, learners will be able to:

- **Distinguish between lobbying and advocacy**
- **Differentiate the roles of stakeholders or interested parties, work groups, task forces, and coalitions in advocacy**
- **Explain how education and advocacy efforts can be used to raise awareness, build consensus and promote health policy, request funding, and lead systemic and environmental changes**
- **Identify strategies to evaluate advocacy efforts**

Keywords

- Advocacy
- Ask
- Consensus Building
- Lobbying
- Request for Proposals (RFP)
- Root Cause
- Stakeholder and Interested Party Analysis Matrix
- Subject Matter Experts (SME)
- Talking Points
- Workgroup

Self-Reflection Question

Take a moment and reflect on these questions:

1. Do you consider yourself to be an advocate? Why or why not?
2. What are indicators of successful advocacy efforts?
3. What if the desired change did not happen? Were the efforts a failure? Why or why not?

DOI: 10.4324/9781003504320-6

Advocacy describes strategic actions to influence and impact policies and procedures at an organizational, community, or systems level. A basic function of advocacy is the act of raising awareness and education. By simply proposing a change in policy or procedure, the opportunity exists to educate individuals or groups. Advocacy is often aimed at policy makers, which can include elected officials, community leaders, and other decision-makers who have a role in voting on and passing legislation, policies, and procedures. When listing the lessons learned about the public health response to COVID-19, public health leaders have expressed how critical it is to be skilled in advocacy. Johns Hopkins Bloomberg School of Public Health (n.d.) leaders reflected on the pandemic saying in part, "We saw firsthand that good science is not good enough. We must intervene in the larger political, economic, and social arenas and more fully engage in advocacy that will lead to programs and policies that protect the public's health" (para. 3). Some have argued that the field of public health stepped away from advocacy over the past few decades by stating:

> Public health has been hobbled by decades of neglect and held back by politics. That is changing. The value of public health has been recognized yet again. We must seize this moment in history and the spotlight on public health's strengths and weaknesses to build the political will to re-envision public health and rebuild our public health systems.
>
> *(Johns Hopkins Bloomberg School of Public Health [JHBSPH], n.d., para. 3)*

One key way to strengthen public health systems and public health efforts in communities and organizations is through advocacy efforts, because "efforts at communication and advocacy [are] critical in making social, cultural, and policy change possible" (JHBSPH, n.d., para. 4). This chapter will focus on the topic of health advocacy to advance public health outcomes and the skills necessary for HES in this important work. This chapter will also describe and provide examples of lobbying and advocacy efforts because HES may be involved with both in their roles.

Lobbying Versus Advocacy

Advocacy is often confused and used interchangeably with **lobbying**. Lobbying involves advocating; however, it also includes very specific actions that set it apart from advocacy. Lobbying includes actions to influence and impact *specific* pieces of legislation, such as asking an elected official to vote in favor of or against a specific bill. Lobbying includes three elements: a decision maker, legislation or a policy that requires a vote, and a specific request about the vote of the decision maker (National Council of Nonprofits [NCN], 2022).

Rules and policies about who can lobby versus advocate can depend on local policies, federal guidelines, and expectations from an employer. For example, organizations that are classified as 501(c)(3) must abide by specific Internal Revenue Services (IRS) regulations in order to retain their classification as a nonprofit. However, the guidelines for lobbying are vague and can cause confusion. Specifically the IRS (2022) states that 501(c)(3) organizations "may engage in some lobbying, but too much lobbying activity risks loss of tax-exempt status" (para. 2). This vague language of the word '*some*' does not clarify the difference between '*some*' and '*not too much.*' This is believed to be why some nonprofit organizations may choose not to engage in any lobbying efforts (NCN, 2022). It may also explain why some professionals are concerned about engaging in lobbying. It is critical for HES to know if they are eligible to lobby within the scope of their jobs and that they are in compliance with policies.

Role of Advocacy

Advocacy is an incredibly powerful tool when done well. Effective advocacy can accomplish each of the following:

- Build relationships with policy makers;
- Educate and influence a policy maker or lawmaker's decision;
- Alter existing policies, laws, and budgets; and
- Encourage the creation of new programs (National Association of County and City Health Official [NACCHO], 2017, p. 2).

The power of advocacy is astounding and incredibly valuable. Advocacy work is also long-term and ongoing. It can also feel like a lot of work is needed for small, yet important, changes to happen. There are no quick and easy victories. Advocacy work is equivalent to running a marathon, as opposed to a sprint. In addition to effective communication, it requires commitment, dedication, and strategic planning to be successful.

The reality is that there are a lot of opportunities to improve health outcomes and raise awareness and implement changes in policies. Therefore, the list of things to advocate for or against is quite lengthy. Advocacy requires patience and perseverance. It relies heavily on building relationships with community members and policy makers. Building these relationships takes time. It takes time to build trust and understand how the topics being advocated fit in the larger context of the community being impacted.

A key component of advocacy is education. In addition to raising awareness among policy makers, education can also raise awareness among community members who would be impacted by a change in policy and why it matters. Education can also result in a deeper understanding among professional staff and volunteers who are engaging in the advocacy work. It is important when delivering education as a component of advocacy that the information is clear, science-based, and simple to understand. Often health topics can be complex. The science may also be limited, which raises many questions, and the concepts being advocated for may overlap with other health topics or behaviors. When delivering education as part of advocacy efforts, it is important to help the policy or decision-maker find the connection between the information that they are learning (or being reminded of) and how the proposed change can be helpful in positively impacting health outcomes. A policy or decision-maker is often well-versed and a subject matter expert in their own area of expertise. However, it is the job of an advocate to educate them on the proposed topic and ensure that they have a solid understanding of how the proposed actions can be helpful or a lack of action might be hurtful.

Effective advocacy can change not just policies and practices but also laws and budgets. A policy change would result in potentially time-limited changes in businesses and organizations at the local, state, or federal level. It may be time limited because it may serve a specific purpose at that time or may be the actions of specific leadership, and when that leadership changes – the policies may no longer be enforced. In comparison, a change to a law would impact the courts, policing, and how governing bodies carry out their duties. Changing a law is a lot more time-consuming and requires different action steps than a policy. Advocacy can also result in a change in budgets because if, for example, a policy or law was modified to require water fountains to be installed at all community parks, then to ensure that this change is implemented funding would need to ensure that the resources are in place to purchase the supplies, ensure water lines are in place, and compensate personnel.

Sometimes advocacy efforts result in a new program or service being developed. This may happen because existing programs and services do not meet the identified need adequately or at all. For example, Live Healthy Miami Gardens was established in 2014 and is a "Collective Impact Initiative bringing people together and strengthening the community's capacity to collaboratively plan and collectively carry out strategies that make the vibrant community of Miami Gardens healthier" (Live Healthy Miami Gardens [LHMG], 2020c, para. 2). One key focus area for the initiative is physical activity, which was identified through surveys and focus groups. The group found that more than half of community members have sedentary jobs and more than a quarter reported not having time for physical activity (LHMG, 2020b). As a result, the group has instituted multiple strategies and programs to support physical activity such as planting over 300 trees "near walking and biking trails and transit stops to promote physical activity and public transit use" and "creating wayfinding signs touting the benefits of walking and biking" with help from over 200 community volunteers (LHMG, 2020a). Although this may not have started as an advocacy project initially, the result has been that the needs of community members were identified and addressed to better the community and the lives of the residents. Having over 200 community members engaged in this planting process is also an incredible statement of the support from the community for this effort.

Who Can Be an Advocate

Anyone can be an advocate and they can do this for any cause or issue. An individual may be an advocate because they are passionate about a particular issue, they may want to raise awareness about an issue, or they may want to promote best practices for addressing it. It may be in a person's job description or position requirement to advocate for specific issues or causes. The audience for the advocacy can vary greatly. Advocacy can occur within friendship circles and family members, within a community, or with elected officials. The elected officials can be local, state, or federal.

Types of Advocacy

Advocacy can also be formal and informal. Informal advocacy may be in the form of encouraging friends and family to shop at the local farmer's market or to compost at home. Informal advocacy is unpaid and not formalized in its approach. It may be sporadic, yet can still have the power to change perceptions and behaviors. It may raise awareness in others and contribute to improving health outcomes overall without a strategic plan. It can include being an advocate for a family member who is hospitalized and should be seen by a specialist or a pet who has been having symptoms and the veterinary staff is not responding urgently. Informal advocacy can include following up with an academic adviser who has not responded to requests for a signature to complete a transfer application. Informal advocacy can be done in many ways, at any time.

Formal advocacy refers to efforts usually led by an organization. For example, the Human Rights Campaign (HRC) is an advocacy organization whose work is centered around campaigns that are "focused on mobilizing those who envision a world strengthened by diversity, where our laws and society treat all people equally, including LGBTQ+ people and those who are multiply marginalized" (n.d., para. 2). Individuals can sign up for updates from HRC to learn about opportunities to sign petitions launched by HRC or join in phone banking efforts to garner support from voters to advance policies that treat people equally.

Activity 6.1: Discussion

Sometimes community members are passionate about health, but engaging with an elected official or demanding change seems intimidating, futile, or overwhelming.

1.   Why do you think community members feel this way?
2.   How could a HES motivate community members to participate in advocacy efforts?

Individual Advocacy

There are many individuals who self-identify as an advocate. Sometimes individuals may be in the role of an advocate and not even realize it. They may simply be participating in the advocacy process because they care about a particular cause and want to see change. Perhaps the individual is advocating for themselves and a health matter that impacts them. Sometimes, individuals believe that informal advocacy is not genuine advocacy or that one individual can't make a difference. That is simply incorrect. Dr. Mary T. Bassett, the former Commission for the New York City Department of Health and Mental Hygiene explains that

> [t]he challenge to improve public health calls for the involvement of everyone, including those outside the health sector. Learning how to engage more effectively with communities is essential for health professionals who wish to create programs and institute policies that measurably improve health and lives.
>
> *(2003, p. 1204).*

There are many ways that an individual can engage in public health advocacy. A common example of individual advocacy is writing a letter to the editor of a newspaper. This form of communication can be an easy opportunity to increase awareness of an issue and alert policy makers of the topic. This is typically a short letter that is clear and concise. Generally, there are specific requirements for submitting these letters, including length and topic. Writing a letter to the editor is a chance to identify recommended actions and offer explanations for them. Since these letters are read by a diverse audience, it is important to provide context on the matter being addressed as some readers may be completely unaware, while others may share your interest and agree. Limiting your message to a few points, with a strong message, may also help to ensure your letter is published (Dorfman, 2015).

Activity 6.2: Practice Your Skills

Identify a public health issue that is important to you. Suppose you were going to write a letter to the editor of a local newspaper or testify before your local City Council.
 Consider the following questions:

1.   What are three pieces of information that you believe are most important to share about this public health issue?
2.   What is the change that you want?
3.   Why do you think this change would make a positive impact?

SIDEBAR: DID YOU KNOW?

Contact information for members of Congress is readily available online. They are also available at the following websites:

■   https://www.congress.gov/members/find-your-member
■   https://www.usa.gov/elected-officials

To learn more about reaching out to elected officials and a sample letter, please visit https://www.center4research.org/writing-policy-makers/

SIDEBAR: DID YOU KNOW?

Sign-on letters or often shared online and publicly available. This is to encourage as many individuals and organizations to add their signatures. To review examples of a sign-on letter, please visit https://www.cfchildren.org/policy-advocacy/joint-advocacy/sign-on-letters/. You can also do a simple internet search for '*sign-on letter*' and a listing of organizations will be provided with the sign-on letters that they have supported.

Individuals may also want to write a letter directly to their elected officials with their advocacy message. Local and state government officials usually have their contact information on a website with an option to submit comments to the office. Individuals can also reach out to their members of Congress directly. The American Public Health Association (APHA) highlights that "[e]ducating your members of Congress about the latest information in the world of public health is critical to ensuring that health-related legislation is based on the most rigorous and current scientific evidence" (n.d.). This means that the implications for individual advocacy are indeed significant.

Writing a letter may be a daunting and intimidating task for some. An alternative may be to sign on to an existing letter. Sometimes an individual or organization takes the lead in authoring a letter to an elected official and then provides the opportunity for others to sign the letter in agreement and in support of the message. This strategy draws on the idea of strength in numbers.

It is common for organizational leaders who represent a group or membership base to sign on to existing letters. They often provide their logo as a visual reference to indicate that their entire body of members has signed on to the letter.

Often an individual's advocacy efforts for themselves provide benefits to others. For example, suppose that an employee recently injured their arm and the injury is preventing them from opening doors easily in the building. Although the Americans with Disabilities Act as amended requires employers to ensure that people with disabilities, whether temporary or permanent, have the same rights and opportunities as everyone else at the workplace, suppose that the buttons to open the doors in a building are not functioning properly (ADA National Network, 2023). The employee may advocate for themselves by going to their Human Resources Department to request that the door buttons be fully operational so that they do not risk further injuring their

> **SIDEBAR: DID YOU KNOW?**
>
> Many national, state, and local organizations with a focus on health topics have a speaker's bureau. Generally, this consists of individuals who are impacted by the topic and volunteer their time to speak to groups about the issue.
>
> The National Alliance on Mental Illness (NAMI) is "dedicated to improving the lives of people with severe mental illnesses" (National Alliance on Mental Health Virginia [NAMIV], 2023, para. 1). There are over 600 state organizations and affiliates that help carry out the work (National Alliance Mental Illness, 2023). NAMI Virginia promotes their speaker's bureau on their website and explains that this bureau includes "lived experience, professional experience, and advanced degrees in public policy, social work, psychology, education or administration" and can present on a wide variety of topics, including advocacy (NAMIV, 2023, para. 1).
>
> To learn more, please visit https://namivirginia.org/speakers-bureau/

arm in their healing process. Although the employee may benefit from this self-advocacy directly, other colleagues and visitors to the premises will also benefit from the door buttons fully functioning.

There are other times when individuals may be interested in advocating for a cause that they may care deeply about for multiple reasons and want to see change for others. These individuals are not necessarily affiliated with a particular organization or group, they may just represent themselves and use their voice to advocate across platforms as an individual. An example of this includes Gavin Grimm's advocacy efforts. Gavin Grimm came out as transgender at his high school in 2014 at the age of 15 (Baska, 2021; Robert F. Kennedy Human Rights [RFKHR], 2022;). Gavin initially received support from his principal who approved his use of the men's restroom until a group of parents complained to the school board. After a public meeting of the school board, which disparaged Gavin, he was banned from using the men's restroom at school (RFKHR, 2022). All Gavin wanted was to "be a normal child and use the restroom in peace" (Wakefield, 2021, para. 1). A legal battle ensued after Gavin sued the Virginia Gloucester County School Board for discrimination (Baska, 2021). Gavin's case went all the way to the Supreme Court. Ultimately, Gavin won his case after the Fourth Circuit Court of Appeals upheld a ruling that the school board "violated both Title IX and the Equal Protection Clause of the Constitution's 14th Amendment" (RFKHR, 2022, para. 2). Advocating for his own rights, ended up also protecting the rights of other transgender youth. Specifically, "the precedent set by the court in Grimm's case covers states that fall within the circuit—Virginia, Maryland, North Carolina, South Carolina, and West Virginia—and will provide a road map for courts elsewhere in future fights over transgender rights" (RFKHR, 2022, para. 3).

Group Advocacy

There are also opportunities for individuals to join organized efforts with other individuals who share similar values to advocate for changes and provide education on issues that matter to them. For example, Everytown is the "largest gun violence prevention organization in America" with nearly 10 million supporters focused on guns in schools, gun suicides, mass shootings, and hate crimes (2022, para. 1). This group of advocates is "building a movement to register voters, elect candidates who will govern with gun safety in mind, demand action from our elected officials, change how Americans think about gun violence, [and] end gun violence" (Everytown, 2022, para. 3). Staff at Everytown mobilize and engage with this group of advocates in strategic ways to advance these goals.

Opportunities also exist at the community level to participate in group advocacy. For example, the disability revolution in the United States was a product of group advocacy.

Activity 6.3: Discussion

For this activity, please watch the documentary *Crip Camp: A disability revolution*. This documentary is available at https://tinyurl.com/367pdpu4 and runs less than 2 hours (CC is available). It describes the movement in the United States to pass federal legislation to protect the rights of people with disabilities and how a summer camp played a pivotal role.

Respond to the following questions:

1. Describe an example of individual and group advocacy that was highlighted in the film.
2. Name one barrier that the advocates faced at the federal level in advancing efforts for equal rights for those with disabilities.
3. What skills did the advocates utilize in their efforts? Why were these skills necessary?

Stakeholders and Interested Parties

The term stakeholders and interested parties are used to describe members of the community, partner organizations, and others who have a vested interest in the community's health. Anyone can be a stakeholder or interested party. These individuals are engaged in assessing the needs of communities and in advocacy efforts. Groups of stakeholders and interested parties can be organized into coalitions, workgroups, and task forces to advocate for policy and systems-level changes to improve health outcomes.

Identifying stakeholders and interested parties to approach and invite into advocacy efforts can be an important strategic move. These individuals can be both impacted by advocacy and could even influence the outcome of advocacy efforts. So considering who these individuals may be and what they are able to contribute can be a helpful activity to engage in. One way to do this is through a **stakeholder and interested party analysis matrix**. This matrix contains several aspects to consider for individual stakeholders. The organization *tools4dev* developed a template that communities and HES can utilize in this process. The document includes the following points for consideration:

■ The name of the stakeholder or interested party and their contact information;
■ The level of impact that the project or advocacy efforts may impact them;
■ The level of influence that they may have over the outcome of the project or advocacy efforts;
■ The most important thing to them about the issue or topic;
■ The specific ways that they can contribute to the project or advocacy effort;
■ The specific ways that they may be a barrier to the success of the project or advocacy effort; and
■ The plan to engage the stakeholder or interested party (tools4dev, 2022).

Being intentional about who to invite in advocacy efforts like this can help avoid potential barriers along the way and also identify possible pathways for success.

Coalition

A coalition describes a collection of individuals and/or groups that are working toward a common goal. Coalitions bring "professional and grass-roots organizations from multiple sectors together, expands resources, focuses on issues of community concern, and achieves better results than any single group could achieve alone" (Society for Public Health Education [SOPHE], 2016, para. 1). The power of a coalition in advocacy is significant. The members are able to bring their expertise and connections to the group to support achieving the common advocacy goal. Coalitions work together to raise awareness, develop and enhance policies, and improve built environments through short- and long-term goals. These advocacy goals could be in a Community Health Improvement plan or be an additional role that they independently have in a community. Coalitions invest significant time and energy in collaborating with community leaders and policy makers to identify and advocate for sustainable and scalable improvements and changes.

There are many reasons why an advocacy coalition may be formed. These can include responding to a funding opportunity or responding to a threat or outbreak (SOPHE, 2016). Communities can receive financial support from government agencies or community organizations through funding opportunities. Typically, this requires completing an application and proposing an idea, the rationale for the idea, an implementation plan, a staffing plan, and a budget. This means that there needs to be an organized response to the funding opportunity. Often funders want to support community coalitions because they have already established collaborative relationships to focus on a common goal and would be better suited to make meaningful and sustainable changes. If a coalition is not already in place, then one may be established to apply for the funding. If awarded the funding, it can be used as a starting point for the work of the coalition to formally begin.

An advocacy coalition may also be formed when there is an immediate need, such as a community threat or outbreak. Knowing that coalitions have multiple aspects of a community represented through individuals and/or organizations this group can help make collaborations run more smoothly since these individuals would connect on a regular basis to focus on the common threat or need. For example, the South Carolina Department of Health and Environmental Control (SCDHEC) encouraged the formation of coalitions in response to the COVID-19 pandemic across the state. These coalitions would be focused on raising awareness on best practices for addressing the pandemic at the local level, sharing data about rates of transmission, and supporting members in implementing response strategies (South Carolina Department of Health and Environmental Control [SCDHEC], n.d.). The SCDHEC offered guidance to local communities on how to establish coalitions. They also encouraged diverse representation to include local government, faith-based leaders, public health organizations, and local businesses (SCDHEC, n.d.).

Coalitions also focus on public health issues that are significant but not an immediate threat like an outbreak, such as eliminating poverty. For example, Mayors for a Guaranteed Income is "a network of mayors advocating for a guaranteed income to ensure that all Americans have an income floor" with over 100 mayors participating (Mayors for a Guaranteed Income [MGI], 2021, para. 10). Guaranteed Income "is a cash payment provided on a regular basis to individuals or households, with no work requirements, and no strings attached. It is intended to create an income floor below which no one can fall and promote the dignity of all" (The Guaranteed Income Pilots Dashboard, n.d.). In 2022, over 30 pilot programs were implemented in cities across the U.S. providing families with cash to spend on groceries, gas, and utilities (MGI, 2022). Most of the Guaranteed Income projects at the local level thus far have received local, state, and federal funding (Holder, 2022). In addition to implementing programs at the local level, MGI and others advocate for state- and federal-level policies and sustained financial support (MGI, 2022).

Workgroup

A workgroup is typically composed of a diverse representation of stakeholders and interested parties with a common goal. A workgroup is sometimes referred to as a working group, a committee, or a sub-committee. Therefore, a workgroup can be included within a coalition or an advisory group. The workgroup is typically tasked with a specific project and meets regularly.

An example of a workgroup at the Maryland Hospital Association (MHA) is a subset of the Behavioral Health Advisory Group (2022). The advisory group is composed of leaders of hospitals and mental health clinicians to advise the MHA on ways that hospitals across the state can support mental health needs (Maryland Hospital Association [MHA], 2022). Within this advisory group are multiple subsets, including a workgroup focused on legislative strategy. This workgroup "is composed of government affair leads that are engaged in advocacy efforts in Annapolis. This group meets monthly during the interim and weekly during the legislative session. This group is critical to strategy development on a myriad of issues affecting the hospital field."

(MHA, 2022, para. 5). Other workgroups focus on topics such as Medicare, liability, and technical support. This workgroup has a long-term commitment to its duties and helps the advisory group address month-to-month needs.

Task Force

Typically, the main difference between a workgroup and a task force is time. A task force is generally composed of a group of stakeholders and interested parties with a specific purpose for a finite amount of time. One example of a task force focused on advocacy is the one developed by White House Executive Order 13995 issued in January 2021 to "provide specific recommendations to the President of the United States for mitigating inequities caused or exacerbated by the COVID-19 pandemic and for preventing such inequities in the future" (U.S. Department of Health and Human Services [HHS], 2022, para. 2). This task force was composed of 12 individuals who were not federal employees and 6 representatives from federal agencies and met eight times to accomplish their goal (HHS, 2022). In addition to the eight meetings of the whole task force, there were sub-committee meetings throughout ten-month span to prepare presentations for the entire task force to identify the final recommendations to provide to the President (HHS, 2022).

SIDEBAR: DID YOU KNOW?

APHA, a leading public health membership organization, engages in public health advocacy through education and campaign efforts. Education efforts include sharing "information about specific issues without the expectation of specific policy action," while campaign efforts are used to "engage the public, members, or target groups to directly encourage policy makers to consider policy action on a specific public health issue" (American Public Health Association, 2022, para. 6–7).

To learn more about APHA, benefits of being a member, and advocacy efforts underway, please visit https://www.apha.org/

Key Components in Advocacy

Successful advocacy requires multiple skills. These skills include understanding the health issue, communicating effectively, building relationships, and managing projects and staff appropriately.

Understanding the Issue

An advocate needs to be knowledgeable about the topic and be prepared to defend the proposed solution. Specifically, advocates need to be able to articulate the following types of information about what they are advocating:

- Information about the health issue (including risk factors, symptoms, treatment options);
- Demographics and statistics on who is impacted and how often, including those disproportionately affected;

- Historical context about what has been done previously to address the issue and why those efforts were or were not successful;
- Which decision-makers have supported efforts on this topic previously or have indicated that they would be open to supporting it and why;
- Which decision has opposed efforts on this topic and why; and
- Examples of similar proposals that have been successful.

Advocates need to demonstrate that they understand the health issue fully. This means that they need to be or become a subject matter expert. **Subject Matter Experts** (or Expertise), abbreviated and often known as SME, refers to acquired knowledge and skills on a particular matter or topic through a combination of education and experience of an individual. Advocates need to be prepared to communicate with others about the topic and be able to respond to questions confidently. Advocates need to make sure that they are up to date on new science that may be released on the issue and communicate about it clearly to diverse audiences. It is equally important for an advocate to know who is most impacted by the health issue, how they are impacted, and why they are impacted disproportionately. The Center for Community Health and Development refers to this as finding the **root cause** of the issue (n.d.). The proposal for action steps needs to be informed by what has already happened in terms of advances in policy or the development of programs and services to address the health topic. This includes knowing who has historically been supportive of the health topic and why. It is equally important to learn what has been attempted in the past and has not worked. What proposals have been turned down previously and why. Learning from these experiences may help to make current and future advocacy efforts about the health topic more successful. There may also be examples of efforts that align with the proposal action steps that received support and are going well. This can help to justify why a similar approach may also be successful in the community. It helps log these pieces of information and consider sharing these with advocates for valuable background and insight.

Communicating Effectively

Advocacy done in person, remotely, or on paper necessitates additional key strategies to effectively and appropriately communicate with diverse audiences. Developing talking points is one example of what HES can do to strengthen their communication skills. A **talking point** is a statement or message that conveys an important piece of information. It is usually a message that is shared no matter who is in the audience. Talking points are statements that represent the content and information that will be consistently used in advocating about the issue. Talking points can be short statements that advocates use multiple times in different formats to express facts about the issue and the proposed action steps. For example, defining the topic or explaining it in a simple way should be done consistently to be effective. The audience may likely memorize some pieces of an advocacy message and repeat it. This repeat of a message can help invite others to join in and tell those listening that the cause has additional supporters.

The words that are chosen in advocacy matter. The message should be clear and avoid phrases with double meaning. The message should be consistent to avoid confusion. The message should also be easy to convey to others. By creating talking points, they serve as a guide to anyone who is speaking about the matter. Sometimes these points are memorized word for word and other times they may be used as a starting point for someone who may be more comfortable with oral communication.

> **Communication**
>
> The topic of communication will be further explored in Chapter 7.

Talking points can also evolve. As the advocacy continues, there may be times when the message needs to be tweaked to acknowledge gains made or additional challenges or obstacles in the way of success. Since advocacy can take years, this is very common.

Making the Advocacy Ask. The proposed solution or request being made is often referred to as the **ask** or the advocacy ask. The advocacy ask is specific and is a necessary component of advocacy. While it may be easy to identify the advocacy ask, such as requesting $300,000 in funding to evaluate the safety of playground space in the city or requesting that language in a proposed policy address the elimination of health disparities, actually verbalizing the request or writing the request may seem more challenging. It may feel too assertive for some to be so forthright in a request. The reality though is that the ask itself is the most important part of advocacy. It is the action that is necessary for change to occur.

Elevator Pitch or Elevator Speech. An elevator pitch or elevator speech describes a brief statement made about a specific health topic. For advocacy efforts, this consists of a 45–90 second statement that could be made to a policy maker or community member during a ride on an elevator together. While it is helpful to envision that this is something reserved to be shared while being on an actual elevator, the reality is that this brief statement may be the only thing that an HES can share with someone in any encounter. It may be the beginning of a future conversation or it may be the only thing a HES may be able to share with an individual or group. The point of the elevator pitch or elevator speech is that HES share easy-to-understand information about the topic, the proposed action steps, and the justification for the action steps.

> **Activity 6.4: Practice Your Skills**
> The National Indian Health Board (NIHB) created a guiding document for developing an elevator speech to raise awareness about public health (PH) accreditation efforts among Tribal Public Health Departments. Accreditation is a formal process completed by health departments to align with recommended best practices and guidelines outlined by national standards (National Indian Health Board, 2018) identifies four components of an elevator speech (Table 6.1).

Table 6.1 Components of an Elevator Speech

Opening statement	This statement draws attention to what is being shared. It may be a statistic, fact, or other important component that stands out about the issue.
Explain the issue	This statement describes the issue in simple terms and explains why it is important to address.
Describe proposed solution	This statement outlines the proposed solution or next action steps.
Concluding statement	This statement can be used to summarize the overall proposal and what the proposed action steps will achieve.

Note: Adapted from "Creating an elevator speech." by NIHB (2018). Retrieved from https://www.nihb.org/docs/04162018/Elevator%20Speech%201.4.18.pdf

Consider a health topic that you care deeply about and draft an elevator speech. Share the speech with a few people and ask them for feedback. Consider asking for feedback on your delivery, the content of your speech, and if you included each component effectively.

To learn more about this guidance, please visit https://www.nihb.org/docs/04162018/Elevator%20Speech%201.4.18.pdf.

Building Relationships

Relationships are a core element of advocacy. Successful relationships are rooted in trust and effective communications. These principles also apply to relationships that are identified and developed through health advocacy. Initiating a relationship with policy makers and elected officials can be intimidating; however, it is important to consider that these individuals often rely on advocates to be an important resource (NACCHO, 2017). Skilled advocates know the issue and its impact on the community. Advocates know the community members who work in these spaces and those who have been directly impacted. NACCHO reminds advocates to be confident (2017). This is because advocates have information and a vision for a better community. Their passion and skill set is invaluable. Building relationships can start by following up with the decision-makers after speaking with them. It is helpful to take notes from the conversation and include points made in follow-up contact (Inclusion NB, n.d.).

Activity 6.5: Discussion
Confidence is a key quality in an advocate. Take a moment and share your responses to the following questions:

1. How can a HES grow their confidence as an advocate?
2. How can a HES help volunteers grow their confidence as an advocate?

Managing Projects and Staff

Since HES will likely be in a leadership and coordinating role when it comes to advocacy efforts, there are key project management and people management skills and techniques that will be helpful. Being able to manage multiple deadlines, tasks, and responsibilities will be necessary. This necessitates keeping detailed trackers of key dates and knowing who is responsible for each task. Ideally, HES are working with coalitions or other volunteer or staff groups that can share the various responsibilities for hosting events, training volunteers and staff, and communicating with decision-makers.

People management describes working with volunteers and staff. This ranges from recruitment to training to delegation to providing feedback for performance improvement. Therefore, HES need to be able to describe various roles for volunteers and staff in the advocacy work and ensure appropriate training is provided. Training may be on the decision-making process, who the key decision-makers are, and what the advocacy goals are. When there are long-term strategies as part of the advocacy work, then the demand for support may vary. There may be periods throughout the year that may require more support. For example, there may be ongoing opportunities to raise awareness and recruit stakeholders to support the work. There may also be a large-scale event, such as a public comment opportunity, where community or organization members may be needed to provide testimony in favor or against policies being considered. Being ready to on-board individuals in a thoughtful and strategic manner will aid in successful advocacy efforts. HES may find themselves often working with other groups (such as coalitions from a neighboring city or an employee resource group at a company) that want to help and be involved. Being able to cultivate relationships across communities, within and across networks, is also valuable when working on advocacy efforts. This may mean that HES attend meetings and networking opportunities outside of their typical scope to identify and build those relationships.

Activity 6.6: Discussion

An important role for HES is to model and teach advocacy skills to others.

1. Which skill or skills do you think is most important to teach first? Why?
2. Describe one way that a HES can teach a community member how to effectively manage an advocacy campaign or project.

Accomplishments through Advocacy

Although the work of advocacy is a long-term commitment with the final desired outcome taking years to achieve, it is important to celebrate all of the successes of this work. There are many accomplishments that result from successful advocacy efforts. Examples of accomplishments can include raising awareness, building consensus and promoting health policy, funding, and systems and environmental change.

Raising Awareness

Raising awareness about a public health issue or topic is important work because without awareness, the likelihood for a change in policies, programs, or services in a community may not occur. There are so many things that can have an impact on health outcomes, it is really impossible for any one person to know them all. Education may be the first step in making change happen.

An example of the power of raising awareness is found in the topic of BPA. BPA, the chemical compound called bisphenol A, has been documented for years as being an endocrine hormone disruptor (also called an EDC). The Endocrine Society analyzed and validated the findings of over 1,800 studies in 2015 that found EDCs are "linked to male and female reproductive disorders, obesity, diabetes, neurological problems, immune and thyroid disorders, osteoporosis, Parkinson's disease, and hormone-related cancers" (2023, para. 9). Given this, the Endocrine Society continues to raise awareness about this topic and supports dissemination of scientific studies with the goal of the development of policies and guidelines on EDC use, marketing, and safety standards (2023).

The Food and Drug Administration (FDA) amended regulations in 2012 and 2013 to align with current practices in manufacturing that discontinued BPA in baby bottles, sippy cups, and packaging of infant formula (2018). In January 2022, a coalition made up of public health and environmental groups requested the FDA limit BPA in all food packaging in a petition (Erickson, 2022). The petition was requested and resubmitted by the coalition in April 2022 (Environmental Working Group [EWG], 2022). By June 2022, the FDA agreed to reassess the risks of BPA based on new scientific evidence included in the petition from the European Food Safety Authority (Crunden & Wittenberg, 2022). This move comes after at least a decade of advocacy work. Although this is an evolving topic, this update is significant when considering the potential impacts of improving health outcomes. Educating the public and policy makers was key. The information shared has always relied on the most up-to-date, scientific information. It is crucial that HES are informed about the evolving scientific updates on the topic that they are advocating about.

Building Consensus and Promoting Health Policy

Another result of effective advocacy is a built consensus to aid in promoting health policy. **Consensus building** describes the process of gaining support and agreement among a group. In terms of health advocacy, this can happen when a group is introduced to the health topic and the advocacy ask and agree. For example, suppose that a small group of neighbors are concerned about the amount of speeding in their community. Recently, a child was critically injured after being hit by a speeding automobile. If this small group of neighbors approaches the official neighborhood board and presents both their argument and advocacy ask as a group, it may demonstrate to the leaders of the neighborhood board that this is a shared concern and one that would be given a higher priority. Having group support to advocate for health policy may influence decision-makers to address the need or address it more quickly. It may help decision-makers understand where community support lies in their actions.

Funding

Advocacy can also result in funding of efforts that have not been funded before or an increase in existing funding. One example of this is the funding of guaranteed income programs. As described earlier in this chapter, Guaranteed Income programs are designed to help individuals out of poverty by providing them with a set amount of funds over a period of time. Sometimes these funds come with certain restrictions such as only using the funds to pay specific bills. Officials in the city of Alexandria, Virginia launched a Guaranteed Income pilot program in 2022 for residents with household income at or below 50% of Area Median Income (AMI) to receive cash payments for two years in the amount of $500 without any conditions (Alexandria Living, 2022). The program, limited to 170 households, cost the city $3 million (Alexandria Living, 2022). This program is a success for the community members, organizations, and city partners who have advocated to address the racial income gap and health equity needs for city residents.

Systems and Environmental Change

Ideally, advocacy efforts can have an impact on root causes. Systems change work

> refers to the process of improving the capacity of a system or group of systems to work with multiple sectors to improve the health status for all people in a defined community Systemic change moves beyond thinking about individuals and individual organizations, single problems and single solutions.
>
> *(Uncommon Solutions, 2018, p. 3)*

One key example of this is the advocacy work on ending the backlog of rape test kits across the country. Through state and federal efforts to raise awareness of this issue, the practice of logging rape test kits is being changed. End the Backlog is an initiative of the Joyful Heart Foundation, an organization formed in 2004 by Mariska Hargita that is committed to transforming "society's response to sexual assault, domestic violence, and child abuse, support survivors' healing, and end this violence forever" (Joyful Heart Foundation, 2022, para. 3). After a sexual assault, a survivor is able to obtain a sexual assault forensic exam that collects evidence from their body of the assault. This evidence is tagged and stored with the idea that it would be reviewed and analyzed. Fingerprints and other DNA evidence would be compared to identify the perpetrator or perpetrators to seek justice. However, for years thousands of test kits sat in storage units. Survivors did not know the status of their kits and perpetrators who had matching DNA available were not held responsible. Often due to a lack of funding, labs across the country did not have the support to process the kits. End the Backlog was an initiative to raise awareness about this issue and change the laws and funding for this issue. In 2014, the Sexual Assault Kit Initiative was introduced and by 2015 a total of 48 law enforcement agencies in 27 states were provided funds to address their backlog (End the Backlog, n.d.).

SIDEBAR: DID YOU KNOW?

To learn more about the policies in place to locate a rape test kit in your state, please visit https://www.endthebacklog.org/information-for-survivors/locating-a-rape-kit/.

Concepts in Action 6.1

Background: José (he/him) works at a local health department and directs the chronic disease prevention efforts. He has worked with multiple coalitions across the city over the past few years. One of the coalitions has worked diligently to identify opportunities to promote healthy eating and active living within the community. One strategy that the coalition supports is healthier vending options. The coalition is interested in proposing mandating healthier vending machines located in City-owned buildings to the City Council. This would include city hall, recreation centers, city offices, and service centers run by the city. In total, there are approximately 132 vending machines that would be impacted. The coalition has turned to José for help navigating the process in the city.

Initially, José looked for guidance on implementing healthy vending. He quickly found guidance from ChangeLab Solutions (2022), an organization with a mission to advance health equity through public health laws and policies, on their website at https://www.changelabsolutions.org/product/making-change-healthier-vending-municipalities.

After reviewing the guidance from ChangeLab Solutions and others, José developed the following plan to guide how he will support the coalition in educating council members on this topic and the proposal for healthy vending.

Over four phases, the proposal to the City Council will be developed and presented to the City Council. Prior to a presentation to the City Council as a whole, the members of the coalition would reach out to the individual members and explain their proposal to build consensus and identify potential opportunities to enhance the proposal prior to being presented to the City Council formally. This interaction is also an opportunity to develop or nurture an existing relationship with the Council members. Prior to presenting to the Council formally, the coalition members will determine who will conduct the formal presentation and prepare them for potential questions from the Council (Table 6.2).

In the development of the proposal, José encouraged the coalition to identify ways that they can offer support to the city in implementing the proposal, as it would be a significant commitment. For example, the coalition should be prepared so that the council may ask them to draft an RFP, also called a **Request for Proposals**, to solicit vendors along with city staff. The solicitation would serve as an application process for a selection committee to identify the vendor that the city would hire to service the vending with healthy food options. Coalition members should also be prepared to have representation in the selection committee to interview applicants and help identify the best vendor. Exploring the various ways for the coalition to support the implementation of a change that they would like to see is a way to also identify strategies for building relationships with elected officials and decision-makers in the city. Successful implementation of this effort may help the coalition in addressing other health needs in the city.

Table 6.2 Phases to Present Proposal to City Council

Phase One	Develop proposal	Research topic and best practices
Phase Two	Contact individual council members	Contact City Council members to explain the proposal
Phase Three	Prepare coalition to present	Describe Council meeting logistics, identify responses to potential questions, practice testimony
Phase Four	Present proposal	Present proposal during testimony

Challenges and Opportunities

Advocacy work is incredibly satisfying work. It can lead to monumental changes that will lead to informed community members and policy makers. This work also comes with multiple challenges and opportunities for HES.

Challenges

Challenges include the capacity that supporters have to participate in advocacy efforts. Whether the majority of supporters are volunteers or professional staff, there are limitations in time and expertise.

Volunteer Commitment Versus Professional Commitment. Because anyone can be an advocate, advocacy efforts can be supported by professional staff and volunteers. Therefore, it is important that HES establish opportunities that can be supported by either group. For example, working with large groups of volunteers is very different from working with professional staff within an organization. Volunteers may or may not have jobs, families, and other commitments that may impact their availability to participate. They may also need specialized training on the topic. Some volunteers may need more advance notice of opportunities to help, while some may be available for immediate needs. Managing this kind of availability requires HES working in advocacy to be able to manage multiple schedules, provide effective communications, exercise flexibility, and strategically engage volunteers.

Professional staff that support advocacy efforts often work for the host organization of the advocacy efforts or a supporting organization that has made a commitment to support the efforts. Professional staff who work full time and are assigned to specific advocacy projects will often have performance expectations in accomplishing specific tasks and have dedicated time to participate in activities. Professional staff, which can include other HES, often have experience and knowledge of advocacy actions and can serve in leadership roles.

Emerging Topics. Since advocates utilize science and evidence-based practices to develop their advocacy ask, it is necessary to maintain up-to-date subject matter expertise on the topics. This requires time and intention to identify relevant and appropriate sources to review on a consistent and regular basis. For example, if the advocacy ask includes a change in policy then staying informed about other communities that have successfully implemented similar policies would be helpful to include in talking points. Scientific advances in technology and analysis of data should also be reviewed to ensure that the advocacy ask contains the most up-to-date information.

Opportunities

Health advocacy also provides opportunities to engage community members and policy makers in important issues and build meaningful relationships. These ongoing relationships can create a network of support for emerging needs and issues.

Engage All Members of the Community. Anyone can be an advocate. Each community or organization that HES work in has stakeholders who are vested in the health outcomes of the members. There are many ways that members of any community can participate in advocacy efforts. From logistical support to actually communicating with decision-makers, the ways to support advocacy efforts are endless. HES should find opportunities to inquire about the ways that community members can and want to be a part of advocacy efforts, what subject matter expertise they bring with them, and what they hope to accomplish. There may be some community members who have more availability and/or interest to be part of this work than others. No matter how much time someone has or what expertise they bring with them, HES should be able to find meaningful ways to engage community members who want to participate. Perhaps if they have a positive experience, they may want to assume greater responsibilities in the next project.

Opportunity for Network of Support. The reality is that communities often share similar health concerns. Certainly, the concerns may change in terms of significance and priority. The types of resources and community assets may also vary across communities. However, it is a similar skill set and passion that is shared among those who work in the health advocacy space. This means that across communities there are opportunities to support other health advocates with resources, ideas, and support. There may even be opportunities for collaboration, such as developing programs across a region.

Eight Areas of Responsibility for CHES® and MCHES®
Advocacy aligns with the following area of responsibility for CHES® and MCHES®.

Area V: Advocacy

This area includes four competencies and 18 sub-competencies for advocating (National Commission for Health and Education Credentialing, Inc. [NCHEC], 2020). This includes identifying a health issue that can be addressed with a policy- or system-level intervention and potential stakeholders to support efforts to raise awareness of the issue and promote changes (NCHEC, 2020). Situational and contextual awareness to promote changes are necessary to achieve proposed changes. This includes understanding how proposed changes may impact the community intentionally and unintentionally. It also includes knowing the current policies, procedures, and practices in place and how a change to these can be accomplished (NCHEC, 2020). Furthermore, this area includes skills such as mobilizing stakeholders and reviewing the effectiveness of the effort to change policies or system-level interventions (NCHEC, 2020).

To learn more about the Areas of Responsibility, please visit https://www.nchec.org.

Evaluation of Advocacy

Effective advocacy requires thoughtful planning and evaluation. It is best to identify an evaluation strategy of advocacy efforts in the planning phase. Evaluating advocacy efforts are necessary to inform future advocacy efforts. As indicated in Table 6.3, evaluation methods for each objective type for an advocacy activity can vary.

Assessing the number of distributed postcards at an event can simply be an inventory count, while determining if volunteers felt that the advocacy training they received was helpful can be evaluated through a survey. While not all advocacy efforts end with the passing of legislation, this is an example of a long-term outcome that is the result of hard work, commitment, and a passion for change.

Table 6.3 **Examples of Advocacy Evaluation Methods**

Objective Type	Objective Example	Evaluation Methods
Process objective	By July 15, distribute at least 1,200 postcards about the health issue at the public health event	Count of the postcards remaining
Impact objective	By October 1, at least 75% of new volunteers as of July 1 will report the phone banking training was helpful or somewhat helpful to make calls to inform registered voters on the health topics included on the upcoming election ballot	Survey of volunteers after they have completed their first week of phone backing
Outcome objective	By 2027, a new policy on healthy food options on campus will be enacted	Review of the policies

Activity 6.7: Practice Your Skills

For each of the following strategies, identify which is *good*, *better*, or *best* in terms of advocacy.

Registering and Voting

_____Encourage your friends and family to vote

_____Volunteer to register members in your community to vote at a local farmer's market

_____Register to vote and vote in each local and national election

Participating in Elections

_____Run for City Council or seek getting an appointed position by an elected official

_____Donate to the campaign of a candidate with a commitment to public health efforts

_____Volunteer to support a candidate committed to public health on their phone bank

Direct Lobbying

_____Submit a letter through a policy maker's website expressing your views on an issue

_____Meet with your elected representative in your state about an issue important to you

_____Develop ongoing relationships with your elected representatives by attending and participating in their town hall meetings and other public events

Integrating Grassroots Lobbying into Direct Lobbying

_____Get on the agenda for an upcoming City Council meeting and provide testimony on an issue that is important to you

_____Start an online petition to advocate a specific policy in your community

_____Organize a coalition in your community to advocate for policy changes to improve health outcomes

Using the Internet

_____Use the internet to search for information on an issue that is important to you

_____Build a website to educate others about ways to address the issue through policy or legislative actions

_____Volunteer to teach others on how to use the internet for effective advocacy efforts

Note: This assignment was adapted from "Advocacy 101: Getting started in health education advocacy." by Galer-Unti, R., Tappe, M., & Lachenmayr, S. (2004). *Health Promotion Practice*, *5*(3), 280–288.

Summary

- Advocacy describes strategic actions to influence and impact policies and procedures at a community, organizational, or systems level. Lobbying involves advocating; however, lobbying includes actions to influence and impact specific pieces of legislation, such as asking an elected official to vote in favor of or against a specific bill.

- Groups of stakeholders and interested parties can be organized into coalitions, workgroups, and task forces to advocate for policy- and systems-level changes to improve health outcomes. Coalition members bring their expertise and connections to the group to support achieving the common advocacy goal. A workgroup is typically tasked with a specific project and meets regularly while a task force is generally composed of a group of stakeholders and interested parties with a specific purpose for a finite amount of time.

- Education and advocacy efforts can be used to raise awareness, build consensus and promote health policy, request funding, and lead systemic and environmental changes.

- It is necessary to plan for evaluations in the planning phase to ensure that advocacy interventions and programs are effective and meet the stated objectives. There are multiple ways to evaluate advocacy efforts. These include determining the number of contacts made or materials distributed, surveys, and whether a policy or procedure was adopted.

Web Resources

- **NACCHO Advocacy Toolkit**

  https://www.naccho.org/uploads/downloadable-resources/2018-gov-advocacy-toolkit.pdf

  The NACCHO Advocacy Toolkit was developed for local public health officials and explores the differences between advocacy and lobbying. Information and tips on engaging with members of Congress and their staff are provided, including links to talking points.

- **Tools4dev**

  https://tools4dev.org/resources/stakeholder-analysis-matrix-template/tools4dev This link provides templates and resources for professionals working in international development. Their resources can also be helpful in health promotion and advocacy efforts. This website provides a link to a stakeholder matrix analysis template that can be tailored for any group interested in this activity.

References

ADA National Network. (2023). *What is the Americans with Disabilities Act (ADA)?* https://adata.org/learn-about-ada

Alexandria Living. (2022, Oct. 24). *Guaranteed Income Pilot Program Applications Now Open.* https://alexandrialivingmagazine.com/news/guaranteed-income-pilot-program-ARISE-Alexandria-VA/#:~:text=The%20program%20will%20provide%20cash,Plan%20Act%20(ARPA)%20dollars

American Public Health Association. (n.d.). *The Power of Advocacy.* https://www.apha.org/-/media/Files/PDF/advocacy/Power_of_Advocacy.ashx

American Public Health Association. (2022). *Get the Facts on Advocacy at APHA.* https://www.apha.org/policies-and-advocacy/advocacy-for-public-health/coming-to-dc/get-the-facts-on-advocacy-at-apha

Baska, M. (2021). *Trans Man Who Took School Bathroom Case All the Way to the Supreme Court Facing Homelessness.* https://www.thepinknews.com/2021/12/31/gavin-grimm-home-gofundme-trans/

Bassett, M.T. (2003). Public health advocacy. *American Journal of Public Health, 93*(8), 1204. https://www.ncbi.nlm.nih.gov/pmc/articles/PMC1447936/pdf/0931204.pdf

Center for Community Health and Development. (n.d.). Chapter 30, Section 3: Understanding the issue. *University of Kansas.* https://ctb.ku.edu/en/table-of-contents/advocacy/advocacy-principles/understand-the-issue/main

ChangeLab Solutions. (2022). *Making Change: Healthier Vending for Municipalities.* https://www.changelabsolutions.org/product/making-change-healthier-vending-municipalities

Crunden & Wittenberg. (2022, June 2). *FDA Agrees to Reassess BPA Risks.* E&E News. https://www.eenews.net/articles/fda-agrees-to-reassess-bpa-risks/

Dorfman, L. (2015). *Tips for Writing Effective Letters to the Editor.* Public Health Institute. https://www.phi.org/thought-leadership/tips-for-writing-effective-letters-to-the-editor/

End the Backlog. (n.d.). *Federal Response.* https://www.endthebacklog.org/public-policy/federal-response/

Endocrine Society. (2023). *Why You Should Care.* https://www.endocrine.org/topics/edc/why-you-should-care

Environmental Working Group. (2022). *FDA Agrees to Renewed Call for Reassessing Health Risks of BPA in Food Packaging.* https://www.ewg.org/news-insights/news/2022/06/fda-agrees-renewed-call-reassessing-health-risks-bpa-food-packaging

Erickson, B.E. (2022, January 31). *US FDA Urged to Limit Bisphenol A in Food Packaging Again.* Chemical & Engineering News. https://cen.acs.org/safety/consumer-safety/US-FDA-urged-limit-bisphenol-A-in-food-packaging-again/100/web/2022/01

Everytown. (2022). *Our Approach.* https://www.everytown.org/about-everytown/#our-approach

Food and Drug Administration. (2018). *Bisphenol A (BPA): Use in Food Contact Application.* https://www.fda.gov/food/food-additives-petitions/bisphenol-bpa-use-food-contact-application

Galer-Unti, R., Tappe, M., & Lachenmayr, S. (2004). Advocacy 101: Getting started in health education advocacy. *Health Promotion Practice, 5*(3), 280–288.

Human Rights Campaign. (n.d.). *Our Work.* https://www.hrc.org/our-work

Holder, S. (2022, September 28). For More Than 20 Guaranteed Income Projects, the Data Is In. *Bloomberg.* https://www.bloomberg.com/news/articles/2022-09-28/for-more-than-20-guaranteed-income-projects-the-data-is-in

Inclusion NB. (n.d.). *Tips for Being an Effective Advocate.* https://nbacl.nb.ca/module-pages/tips-for-being-an-effective-advocate/

Internal Revenue Service. (2022). *Lobbying.* https://www.irs.gov/charities-non-profits/lobbying

Johns Hokins Bloomerg School of Public Health. (n.d.) *The Power of Advocacy.* https://publichealth.jhu.edu/about/our-strategic-priorities/advocacy

Joyful Heart Foundation. (2022). *Our Story.* https://www.joyfulheartfoundation.org/about-us/our-story

Live Healthy Miami Gardens. (2020a) *Accomplishments to Date.* http://livehealthymiamigardens.com/physical-activity/

Live Healthy Miami Gardens. (2020b). *Overview.* http://livehealthymiamigardens.com/physical-activity/

Live Healthy Miami Gardens. (2020c). *What Is Live Healthy Miami Gardens?* http://livehealthymiamigardens.com/

Maryland Hospital Association. (2022). *MHA Work Groups and Task Forces.* https://www.mhaonline.org/about-mha/mha-work-groups-and-task-forces

Mayors for a Guaranteed Income. (2021). *About Us.* https://www.mayorsforagi.org/about

Mayors for a Guaranteed Income. (2022). *End of Year Report 2022.* https://static1.squarespace.com/static/60ae8e339f75051fd95f792e/t/63a4a6119e99192e4dee690b/1671734802641/MGI_End+of+Year+Report_2022_FINAL+DIGITAL+%281%29.pdf

National Alliance on Mental Illness. (2023). *Find Your Local NAMI.* https://www.nami.org/findsupport

National Alliance Mental Illness Virginia. (2023). *Speakers Bureau.* https://namivirginia.org/support-and-education/presentations/speakers-bureau/

National Association of County and City Health Officials. (2017). *The NACCHO Advocacy Toolkit.* https://www.naccho.org/uploads/downloadable-resources/2018-gov-advocacy-toolkit.pdf

National Commission for Health and Education Credentialing, Inc. (2020). *Areas of Responsibility, Competencies and Sub-competencies for Health Education Specialist Practice Analysis II 2020 (HESPA II 2020).* https://assets.speakcdn.com/assets/2251/hespa_competencies_and_sub-competencies_052020.pdf

National Council of Nonprofits. (2023). *Let's Get this Straight: Advocacy vs. Lobbying.* https://www.councilofnonprofits.org/articles/lets-get-straight-advocacy-vs-lobbying#:~:text=%E2%80%9CLobbying%20is%20a%20form%20of,at%20all%20levels%20of%20government

National Indian Health Board. (2018). *Creating an Elevator Speech.* https://www.nihb.org/docs/04162018/Elevator%20Speech%201.4.18.pdf

Robert F. Kennedy Human Rights. (2022). *Gavin Grimm.* https://rfkhumanrights.org/gavin-grimm

Society for Public Health Education. (2016). *Coalition Guide Resource.* https://www.sophe.org/wp-content/uploads/2016/10/Full-Resource-Guide.pdf

South Carolina Department of Health and Environmental Control. (n.d.). *Guidance for Building and Maintaining a Community Coalition.* https://scdhec.gov/sites/default/files/media/document/COVID%20Community%20Coalition%20Guidance%20Doc.pdf

The Guaranteed Income Pilots Dashboard. (n.d.). *About the Dashboard.* https://guaranteedincome.us/about

tools4dev. (2022). *Stakeholder Analysis Matrix Template.* https://tools4dev.org/resources/stakeholder-analysis-matrix-template/

Uncommon Solutions. (2018). *The Guidebook to Successful Policy and Systems Change.* https://kingcounty.gov/depts/health/marijuana-health/~/media/depts/health/marijuana/guidebook_to_successful_policy_and_systems_change.ashx

U.S. Department of Health and Human Services. (2022). *Health Equity Task Force.* Office of Minority Health. https://www.minorityhealth.hhs.gov/omh/browse.aspx?lvl=2&lvlid=100

Wakefield, L. (2021). *Trans Man Wins $1.3m Payout from School that Banned Him from Using Correct Bathroom.* https://www.thepinknews.com/2021/08/26/gavin-grimm-trans-bathroom-case-virginia/?_gl=1*qjgzyq*_ga*MzY1MTMzMTcxLjE2NzQzNTMzNDE.*_ga_BX9CRJ4BBP*MTY3NDM1MzM0Ni4xLjEuMTY3NDM1MzQ2Ny42MC4wLjA

CHAPTER 7

Communicating: Sharing Information Effectively

Keywords

- Cultural Competency
- Health Communication
- Health Communication Campaign
- Health Communication Channel
- Health Equity
- Health Literacy
- Refining
- Segmentation
- Tailoring
- Target Audience

Self-Reflection Questions

Think about an advertisement or campaign about health that you have seen or heard. Perhaps it was a reminder to wear your seatbelt, get a seasonal vaccine, eat five fruits and vegetables each day, or wash your hands.

1. Where were you and what were you doing when you saw or heard this advertisement or campaign?

DOI: 10.4324/9781003504320-7

2. Did you think the message applied to you? Why or why not?
3. Did you change your behavior because of the message that was shared? Why or why not?

Health communication is a complex topic that includes everything from developing messages, to analyzing channels, to choosing platforms to deliver the message. Health communication is an important component of public health. HES use health communication strategies to disseminate information and promote healthy behaviors and lifestyles. Effective health communication is essential for the prevention of diseases, management of chronic conditions, and the overall well-being of individuals and communities. While printed materials were the main method of disseminating health messages in the past, electronic methods, such as social media and screened devices, now dominate how individuals consume all types of information, including health-related content. It is not sufficient to merely create a health message, send it out, and hope it reaches the intended audience. Effective health communication efforts must follow a planned, strategic process (Centers for Disease Control and Prevention [CDC], 2022b). Effective health communication messages and campaigns are successful at changing behavior to improve health because they are focused, tested, evaluated, and improved over time. This chapter will describe the purpose, methods, and skills needed by HES to effectively use health communication strategies to improve individual and community health.

Eight Areas of Responsibility for CHES® and MCHES®
Effectively choosing, delivering, and evaluating health communication messages align with the following Areas of Responsibility for CHES® and MCHES®.

Area VI: Communication

This Area includes six competencies and 26 sub-competencies for creating effective health communication messaging (National Commission for Health and Education Credentialing, Inc. [NCHEC], 2020). This includes using communication models and theories to develop messages for a target audience, examining factors that affect how health messages are received, developing objectives for a health communication campaign, and ultimately developing, selecting, delivering, and evaluating health communication strategies (NCHEC, 2020).

To learn more about the Areas of Responsibility, please visit https://www.nchec.org.

Purpose of Health Communication
The primary purpose of health communication is to encourage the adoption of a healthier behavior or the cessation of an unhealthy behavior. This might include quitting or reducing smoking or drinking alcohol, increasing physical activity, initiating and continuing breastfeeding, reducing screen time, eating a healthier diet, and wearing a face mask in public. A **health communication campaign** is sometimes called a health awareness campaign. However, this term is misleading because it implies that the goal of a health communication campaign is simply to share knowledge. The goal for an effective health communication campaign is to influence a change in behavior.

This can include sharing knowledge on the health topic for the purpose of changing attitudes, beliefs, and perceptions. To influence a change in behavior, the health communication campaign may also include information on how to change the behavior and why it is important to make a change. Health campaigns are designed to "…[educate] individuals and communities about risks and symptoms that may lead to serious health conditions" (Communications Strategy Group, 2023, para. 2). This includes informing individuals and communities about the prevention and management of diseases as well as how to find appropriate healthcare and other resources when needed. The goal is that by having accurate information about current and potential health conditions, people are empowered to seek the education and care they desire.

Key Components of a Successful Health Communications Campaign

Effective health communication campaigns include scientifically accurate information on the health topic using relevant data, recommendations for action, and available resources that are developed for a **target audience** (indicated in Table 7.1).

First, campaigns must provide accurate and authoritative information (Communications Strategy Group, 2023). If a health campaign does not provide fact-based and useful information, they will lose their target audience's attention thus negating the potential positive effects of the effort. Second, sharing actions people can take to prevent a disease as well as what they can do if they are newly diagnosed is important. People generally want action steps they believe they can do to protect themselves and their loved ones. This involves providing timely, relevant, and useful resources and education on the topic. Third, it is important to establish credibility. This cannot be understated. An important reminder for public health professionals during COVID-19 was that medical mistrust can negatively impact health outcomes (Allen et al., 2022). Public health professionals must establish credibility early in a campaign and then maintain it throughout. The fourth component of a successful health campaign is to use current and relevant data as the foundation of the effort. There is a significant amount of data and scientifically accurate information that is readily available at the local, state, and national levels from trusted sources, such as the CDC, for HES to incorporate into a campaign.

For example, if the purpose of a health communication campaign is to decrease the number of adults who are smoking, then the target audience might be adult smokers between the ages of 45 and 64 since this is the age group with the highest smoking rate (CDC, 2023a). Information from credible sources on the impact of tobacco and resources to support adults in this age range on how to quit will need to be identified. If this campaign was aimed at adults between 45 and 64 in a specific county, then the local health department may fund and provide the HES staff to develop and implement

Table 7.1 Key Components in a Successful Health Communication Campaign

Key Components in a Successful Health Communication Campaign	
Accurate information	Credible
Appropriate action items	Current and relevant data

Note: Adapted from "The Importance of Health Awareness Campaigns" by Communications Strategy Group. (2023). Retrieved from https://wearecsg.com/blog/importance-of-health-awareness-campaigns/

the campaign. If this campaign was being developed to target adults between 45 and 64 across the state, then a large-scale campaign might be utilized to reach all counties.

Health Communication Channels

Health communication campaigns use some of the same strategies used in the business and marketing sectors. The difference is that instead of persuading the purchase of a product, health communication campaigns try to persuade the adoption of healthier behaviors and a change in knowledge, attitudes, and beliefs (Communications Strategy Group, 2023). There are many **health communication channels** that HES may use to disseminate health campaigns including, but not limited to, mass media, small media, and social media (Guide to Community Preventive Services [GCPS], 2010). Mass media examples include television, videos, billboards, and radio; small media examples include brochures, fact sheets, infographics, and posters; and social media examples include platforms like Instagram and Facebook (GCPS, 2010). In addition, small and large group sessions are an additional channel HES can use to disseminate health information (GCPS, 2010).

> **SIDEBAR: DID YOU KNOW?**
>
> The Community Preventive Services Task Force recommends the distribution of free or low-cost health-related products as part of a multimedia campaign because campaigns that include both have been effective in changing behaviors (GCPS, 2022). This can include offering free or reduced child safety seats as part of a campaign on safe driving.
>
> To learn more about this recommendation, please visit https://www.thecommunityguide.org/news/new-publications-show-health-communication-works.html

Multimedia

Multimedia campaigns tend to be large in scope and may utilize a combination of communication channels. This might include concurrent messages on cable and streaming, radio, social media, public transit, and print. While multimedia campaigns can be expensive to air, they can be an efficient strategy to promote healthy behavior change to a large audience. These types of campaigns are thoughtfully planned and executed by HES and other public health professionals to encourage behavior change on a large scale. One example of this is the *CDC Tips from Former Smokers Campaign*. This campaign utilizes social media, videos, feature articles, images, and print advertisements and has successfully persuaded over 1 million people to quit smoking since 2012 (CDC, 2023b; Murphy-Hoefer et al., 2020).

> **SIDEBAR: DID YOU KNOW?**
>
> The website for CDC Tips from Former Smokers Campaign provides campaign promotional materials, resources on quitting smoking, and information for specific target audiences on quitting.
>
> To learn more about the campaign, please visit https://www.cdc.gov/tobacco/campaign/tips/index.html

Television and Radio

Sharing health messages or campaigns on television and radio is a common strategy and does not always have to be a part of a multimedia campaign. A message or series of messages may just run as part of a focused campaign.

Since network, cable, and streaming services are now available to most households, television offers an opportunity to reach large numbers of people. There is extensive research on who is watching which television channels and streaming services. For example, because of the relatively high cost of cable, older adults in higher income brackets tend to watch cable (Tvscientific, 2023). However, the percentage of adults watching cable television has decreased from 76% in 2015 to 56% in 2021 (Tvscientific, 2023, para. 7). This type of readily available data can assist HES in choosing specific television stations or streaming services that would be most appropriate for their target audience. There is similar data available about radio listeners (Adgate, 2023).

Public Spaces and Transit

Outdoor and public spaces also offer the opportunity for health campaigns to reach large numbers of people. It is very common to see health communication messages at parks, sports stadiums, and inside buses, trains, stations, and bus shelters. Messages can be included on vinyl banners, posters, flyers, and decals displayed in highly visible locations. Electronic signs are also used to help spread messages in large venues. For example, electronic signs along highways often have messages about speeding, wearing a seatbelt, and driving under the influence. Large billboards are also used along highways and within some large city limits. Although these can be expensive, they can be easily modified with new messages and can be used for multiple campaigns throughout the year.

Telephone and Cell Phones

Receiving health information as recorded telephone messages and text messages to cell phones is very common. Schools, worksites, and communities frequently use these methods to share information about emergencies, but these channels can also be used to share important health information and as part of a health campaign. Pharmacies and healthcare providers often use text messaging to remind people of appointments, when prescriptions are ready for pickup, and the availability of seasonal vaccines. People usually have to opt in to text messaging services, but they can be very effective and inexpensive to administer. Many state tobacco quit phone lines offer a texting service to help people quit smoking. Other companies, such as insurance providers and health-related businesses, use text messaging to deliver reminders about exercising, eating healthy, and managing stress.

Print

Although more and more people rely on social media for information on a wide variety of topics in their life, including health, and entertainment, print media is still relevant, particularly for specific audiences. Print messages appear in newspapers, magazines, newsletters,

> **SIDEBAR: DID YOU KNOW?**
>
> The CDC Office on Smoking and Health and the National Cancer Institute developed the *SmokefreeTXT* program. This is a free service (individual data rates may apply, accessed through the National Texting Portal, that provides six to eight weeks of daily tips, messages to support quitting, and 24/7 support to adults over the age of 18 in the United States who are trying to quit using tobacco.
>
> To learn more about the campaign, please visit: https://www.cdc.gov/tobacco/campaign/tips/quit-smoking/national-texting-portal.html

and bulletin boards located in community centers, laundry facilities, and grocery stores. Flyers are distributed in stores, community centers, worksites and schools, healthcare facilities, and faith-based organizations of varying sizes, ranging from business cards to letter-size sheets of paper. Print health messages might appear on stickers and other paper items. Although not as common or popular as it once was, print media is still incredibly relevant and unlikely to be eliminated as a communication channel despite advances in technology

Social Media and Internet

Finally, any successful health communication effort today must include social media. The target audience will determine which social media platform(s) is chosen. For example, a message designed to reach older adults might be best delivered on Facebook while a message designed to reach college students might be most successful on Instagram, TikTok, or another new and emerging platform that has garnered popularity (Pew Research Center, 2021). There is significant research on social media usage and the data can be stratified by age, income, level of education, ethnicity, and geographic location. Because social media is an ever-evolving landscape, this usage data may change frequently but still offers incredible insight to identify important information on a target audience. Messaging can also be found on the internet when working, shopping, or reading online through targeted advertisements based on internet searches and related cookie data. Messages can also be directed at individuals through emails. Email lists are incredibly valuable because they can contain contact information for hundreds to thousands of individuals. With one email, a significant number of individuals may be reached.

Activity 7.1: Practice Your Skills

CDC's *Hear Her* campaign is designed to increase awareness of urgent maternal warning signs during and after pregnancy and improve communication between patients and their healthcare providers. The goals of the campaign are to:

■ Increase awareness of serious pregnancy-related complications and their warning signs.
■ Empower people who are pregnant and postpartum to speak up and raise concerns.
■ Encourage support systems to engage in important conversations.
■ Provide tools for pregnant and postpartum people and healthcare professionals to better engage in life-saving conversations (CDC, 2022a, para. 4).

Review the campaign's website, https://www.cdc.gov/hearher/index.html to learn more about the campaign and discuss the following questions:

1. Who is the target audience for the campaign? (*Hint*: there are three target groups.)
2. What are the main campaign messages? How do you know this?
3. What are the expected health outcomes associated with this campaign?
4. How will the CDC be able to determine if this campaign is successful?

Health Communication Strategies for Target Audiences

When designing health communication messages, it is important to consider the target audience. Characteristics of the target audience will dictate what messages are used, where they are shared, and how likely they are to be positively received.

Segmentation of the target audience is a strategy that narrows the focus of a health communication campaign to specific groups. For example, HES might develop a campaign to reduce chew tobacco use by teen males with strategies that focus specifically on rural teens as opposed to urban teens. The target audience may be further narrowed to only include males between 10 and 18 who live in rural zip codes within a state. HES can segment their audiences by many factors, including age, gender, and geographic location. By narrowing a target audience into segments, HES can focus their efforts and resources on the specific health behaviors of a smaller group. This strategy is designed to improve the efficiency and effectiveness of limited resources and to develop direct health messages. Therefore, segmentation allows HES to develop and deliver specific health messaging to a specific group of people at a specific time, increasing the likelihood of connecting with the audience and achieving the desired health outcomes.

In addition to audience segmentation, **tailoring** a message involves developing health content for a specific target audience. Tailored messages are designed to appeal to the unique behaviors and attitudes of the group. By tailoring messages, HES can develop a health communication campaign that resonates with the target audience, leading to higher engagement and hopefully the desired behavior change. It can also demonstrate a genuine understanding of the target audience, which can help to build trust. The process of tailoring a message often involves considering factors such as demographics, cultural differences, and even the current health behaviors of the group. For example, a message aimed at teen dating is not likely to be effective for the vast majority of older adults in dating relationships. The images in the campaign will be of young people and older adults would be less likely to connect with the message. Tailoring health messages is an effective way to ensure that health messages make an emotional connection with the target audience, ultimately changing behavior.

Refining health communication messages allows for changes to be made to the message and campaign components so that they are more effective. Refining involves continuous assessment, adjustment, and improvement of the campaign to ensure that the target audience receives it in ways the HES intended. HES will often test or pilot a message on a small segment of the target audience in the refinement process. For example, if a community-wide campaign on increasing physical activity is being developed, project staff might invite five to ten members of the target audience to view and provide feedback on the messages. In this case, different messages may be needed for different age groups or segments of the target audience. Once the campaign launches, further feedback may be solicited to revise the campaign to make it more clear, compelling, and relevant. Refining might include revising the text, changing the graphics or colors used, or changing the tone and style.

Cultural Competence and Health Literacy

Regardless of the methods and channels HES choose for a health communication campaign, two important concepts that must be considered include **cultural competency** and **health literacy**. Cultural competency refers to ensuring that the culture, values, and beliefs of an audience are recognized and honored, regardless if these are different from one's own. The United States is incredibly diverse and this needs to be valued, honored, and represented in health communication activities. For example, health campaigns need to include respectful and accurate representation in language, attire, cultural practices, foods, and faith-based observances and activities. This includes being knowledgeable about significant holidays and observances for various religions. Developing culturally appropriate materials is important, expected, and the right thing to do. HES have a duty to incorporate cultural competency in an effort to help improve access to health information, health services, and community programs that collectively improve health for all. When health information is delivered in a culturally sensitive and respectful manner, the chances of people paying attention and following the messages increase.

One specific way to do this is to tailor interventions and programs based on the culture, values, and language preferences of the target audience. Developing health communication campaigns need intentional design and planning and this can be informed by including members of the target audience in developing campaign content and soliciting their feedback and insight and edits are made. By respecting and recognizing differences in the health beliefs, behaviors, and needs of diverse groups, HES can work toward the goal of eliminating health disparities.

Health literacy refers to the ability of someone to read, comprehend, and act on health information, medical directions, and advice as related to their own health status. About 54% of U.S. adults have a literacy rate below the sixth-grade level, while 79% are considered literate (U.S. Department of Education, 2017). Health literacy includes being able to understand and act on health directives, such as directions on how and when to inject insulin for a person with diabetes; how and when to take a prescribed medication; and, how to safely exercise or when to schedule a follow-up medical appointment. Health literacy is necessary when researching and finding high-quality and accurate health information online. Health literacy is an important skill in improving and maintaining health that many may not have, HES need to be prepared to adapt or tailor intervention materials to also address health literacy.

Health literacy can empower people to improve their health by helping them to understand health education and promotion guidance and recommendations; navigate health and community resources available to them; and make decisions for themselves and their families. For example, if an HES shares the benefits of breastfeeding and offers a

---

SIDEBAR: DID YOU KNOW?

When HES are creating health messages, they must consider using a reading level that the majority of people will be able to comprehend. Communicating a variety of health messages to different target audiences can be challenging. Bakerjian suggests that "...materials should be at a 4th to 6th grade level, use short sentences and simple words, provide evidence-based instructions, and include pictures" (2023, para. 6). The Agency for Healthcare Research and Quality (AHRQ) has a tool, called the Patient Education Assessment Tool, to assess already developed patient education materials. To review the tool, please visit https://www.ahrq.gov/health-literacy/patient-education/pemat.html.

To learn more about creating simple, clear health communication messages, please visit https://www.cdc.gov/health-literacy/pdf/simply_put.pdf.

brochure with examples of the benefits compared to formula feeding to a pregnant person but they do not understand the information being presented, then it is unlikely that they may even consider breastfeeding after the baby is born. This lack of understanding can be because of low literacy, limited reading comprehension, and because of cultural practices in their home that do not support breastfeeding. By taking the time to understand the target audience, listening to the concerns of individuals and addressing them in health communication efforts, and providing accurate and credible information HES and other public health professionals can use health communication messages to improve health.

> ## SIDEBAR: DID YOU KNOW?
>
> The CDC Health Communication Gateway website provides examples of tools available for HES, including campaign examples and templates. Please visit https://www.cdc.gov/healthcommunication/index.html to explore this comprehensive website.

Activity 7.2: Discussion

The National Institutes of Health list several public health campaigns on their website at https://prevention.nih.gov/research-priorities/dissemination-implementation/nih-public-health-campaigns. These campaigns address topics such as brain and heart health, kidney and lung disease, physical activity, tobacco use, and nutrition.

Choose one of the health campaigns listed, review the information provided, and answer the following questions:

1. What is the primary message of the campaign?
2. What communication methods and strategies were used to disseminate the message?
3. Who is the target audience? How do you know?
4. Review the campaign materials. Do you think the creators considered cultural competency when they designed these? Why or why not?

HES must promote **health equity** in all phases of their work, including health communication campaigns. By putting health equity at the center, it underscores the need to be inclusive, respectful, and purposeful when designing health communication strategies. Health equity in health communication means addressing social determinants of health, the impact of racism on health outcomes, and health disparities. To help HES do this, CDC has developed guiding principles "...to help public health professionals, particularly health communicators, within and outside of CDC ensure their communication products and strategies adapt to the specific cultural, linguistic, environmental, and historical situation of each population or audience of focus" (CDC, 2023c, para. 3).

CDC strongly encourages public health professionals and partners in every type of role and at every community at all levels to apply these five overarching principles across their public health communication work, including when creating information resources and presentations, when engaging with partners, and when developing and reviewing external or internal communication materials. These Guiding Principles include:

SIDEBAR: DID YOU KNOW?

Crisis and Emergency Risk Communication (CERC) is a specialized area of health communication (CDC, 2018). Public health professionals who are interested in health communication, perhaps by serving as an agency's Public Information Officer (PIO), can take advanced training offered by the CDC to understand and learn about communicating with the public during a health crisis or emergency. This specialized training includes how a crisis affects people, how to develop messages for different audiences, how to engage the local community, how to manage crisis messages and the media, the different roles of partners at the local, state, and federal levels, and much more.

A wallet card was developed by the CDC to assist public health communicators in times of crisis with tips on how to prepare and respond to questions. To view the card, please visit https://emergency.cdc.gov/cerc/resources/pdf/cerc_wallet-card_english.pdf

To learn more about this specialization, please review the CDC CERC manual at: https://emergency.cdc.gov/cerc/manual/index.asp. For more information on crisis communication and examples of a crisis communication plan, please visit https://ruralhealth.und.edu/communication/crisis.

- *Using a health equity lens* when framing information about health disparities.
- Considering the *key principles*, such as using person-first language and avoiding unintentional blaming.
- Using *preferred terms* for select population groups while recognizing that there isn't always agreement on these terms.
- Considering *how communications are developed* and look for ways to develop more inclusive health communications products.
- Exploring *other resources and references* related to health equity communications (CDC, 2023c, para. 5).

Health equity in health communication includes acknowledging and addressing the social determinants of health, such as income, education, and access to healthcare. This requires creating messages with content that are meaningful to the target audience. If the messages do not resonate with the target audience, then they will be ineffective. HES must be informed about the health topic and the challenges that the target audience is facing. For example, instead of a message that promotes vaccines, consider if the target population has health insurance that will cover the vaccine or if the campaign needs to promote where a free vaccine is available. HES must ensure that health communication campaigns are inclusive, accessible, and culturally sensitive, to promote health equity, decrease health disparities, and improve health outcomes for all individuals, regardless of their background or circumstances. This requires being familiar with translation services available to develop materials in multiple languages, using images that represent different races, religions, gender identities, and abilities. Campaigns must not be used to perpetuate stereotypes or misinformation.

SIDEBAR: DID YOU KNOW?

The National Action Plan to Improve Health Literacy provides a blueprint to improve health literacy and calls for all sectors involved in developing and disseminating health information and services to:

- Provides everyone access to accurate, actionable health information;
- Delivers person-centered health information and services; and
- Supports life-long learning and skills to promote good health (USDHHS, 2010).

The blueprint includes seven goals:

1. Develop and disseminate health and safety information that is accurate, accessible, and actionable
2. Promote changes in the healthcare delivery system that improve information, communication, informed decision-making, and access to health services
3. Incorporate accurate and standards-based health and developmentally appropriate health and science information and curricula into child care and education through the university level
4. Support and expand local efforts to provide adult education, English-language instruction, and culturally and linguistically appropriate health information services in the community
5. Build partnerships, develop guidance, and change policies
6. Increase basic research and the development, implementation, and evaluation of practices and interventions to improve health literacy
7. Increase the dissemination and use of evidence-based health literacy practices and interventions (U.S. Department of Health and Human Services, 2010, para. 2).

To learn more about the National Plan, please visit https://health.gov/our-work/national-health-initiatives/health-literacy/national-action-plan-improve-health-literacy

Activity 7.3: Practice Your Skills

Imagine that you have been asked to create a health communications campaign to encourage children in the community to walk and bike to school. You know that the messages need to reach the parents across the entire school district, focus on the benefits of physical activity for children, and any safety concerns associated with walking and biking routes that have been established. After doing some research on your target audience's demographics, you realize that there are over 15 languages spoken.

Thinking about the goals of the National Action Plan to Improve Health Literacy, consider your response to the following questions:

1. What would you need to consider when creating your messages?
2. What additional issues or concerns should you address?
3. What specific message will be included in the campaign message?
4. What credible sources can be used to ensure the information is accurate?
5. Which invested partners can you ask for help to ensure the messages are person-centered and appropriate given the number of languages spoken?
6. How might the schools participate and contribute to the effort?

Health Communication Evaluation

Evaluating health communications campaigns is a necessary step to ensure the effectiveness of the campaign and its ability to resonate with the target audience. The message needs to also align with the mission, vision, goals, and objectives of the campaign. Most importantly, evaluations assess the clarity and simplicity of the campaign message to determine if it's easy to understand and remember. Being able to remember a message helps to ensure that individuals can implement the recommended actions included in the campaign.

> **SIDEBAR: DID YOU KNOW?**
>
> The CDC has a Public Health Media Library that provides free health-related media for the public. The library includes graphics, websites, apps, and social media content on a wide variety of health topics.
>
> To explore the library and learn more about what it includes, please visit https://tools.cdc.gov/medialibrary/index.aspx#/results.

HES can utilize a variety of methods of evaluation. For example, a focus group may be helpful in determining if the message is clear and memorable. HES may want feedback on the ability of the campaign message to evoke emotions, because emotional appeal can have a profound impact on behavior change. Feedback collected from surveys or focus groups composed of members from the target audience on different versions of campaign materials is another essential tool in the evaluation process to help HES measure the potential impact of the message and make necessary adjustments based on real-world responses. Ultimately, the success of a health campaign can be measured by its ability to achieve desired actions, such as increased awareness, an increase in calls to a hotline, or an increase in the use of public transportation. Regular and thorough evaluation provides HES with the insight necessary to refine and optimize their messages to achieve the campaign goals and continually improve their communication strategies.

Activity 7.4: Practice Your Skills

The CDC's website promotes the health campaign, *Physical Activity. The Arthritis Pain Reliever* at: https://www.cdc.gov/arthritis/interventions/campaigns/physical/overview.htm.

Review the website and campaign materials and consider the following questions:

1. What are the campaign's goals?
2. Who is the target audience?

Next, review the template and example for how to evaluate the reach of a health communication campaign at: https://www.cdc.gov/arthritis/interventions/campaigns/physical/pdf/campaign_reach_template_and_example.pdf.

After reviewing the example provided on pages 2–4, think about how you might implement a similar campaign in your own community.

1. What communication channels would work? Why?
2. What strategies would you use to reach the target audience?
3. Are there channels missing from the example that you think you would add if you implemented a similar campaign? What channels would you include and why?

Communication Skills Utilized by HES

Effective oral and written communication skills are essential for HES to disseminate important health information and promote positive behavioral change in individuals and communities. HES must have the verbal and writing skills to convey at times complex public health messages in a clear and understandable manner, tailoring their messages to diverse target audiences. In addition to being culturally inclusive, HES need to be willing to adapt their communication style to different cultural backgrounds, ensuring their messages are effective with diverse populations without hesitation. Thus, strong interpersonal skills are essential for building rapport and facilitating open, non-judgmental dialogues, especially when addressing sensitive health topics, such as sexually transmitted infections.

HES often give presentations to organizations, worksites, community groups, or elected officials, such as a city council or board of health. HES also present on podcasts videos. In most cases, PowerPoint slides or similar programs are used to create the presentation. Presentations need to be accessible and include Closed Captions, sign language interpretation, and translations when requested. Closed Captions are helpful for audience members for a variety of reasons. Audience members who are hard of hearing or deaf will rely on these, but these can also be helpful for those who may be watching a recording of a presentation and prefer to read along or can't play the audio. Closed captions are also helpful for neurodivergent learners. There are recommended standards and recommendations for formatting to use when creating presentations (Naegle, 2021). These include having no more than six bullet points per slide in a font size that is legible by those in the back of the room, speaking about each slide for approximately one to two minutes, listing the amount of content on each slide, and providing references and sources for the content that is shared. To give an engaging presentation, HES must also have excellent oral skills. Public speaking is a skill that requires practice, practice, and then more practice.

Written communication is perhaps the most used strategy because it can be used alone and in conjunction with other strategies, such as text included in a video. Written communication also included social media posts and blogs. HES may use social media to share information about where programs and services are being held, steps people need to take during an emergency, or general information about a health topic, such as Breast Cancer Awareness Month. Using correct grammar, spelling, and complete references is important. HES often collaborate with colleagues to proofread each other's work, regardless of how long they have been in their role. Maintaining credibility is key and all written work needs to be of the highest quality. This requires being open to feedback and making edits, as needed.

Concept in Action 7.1

Background: *Aisha* (she/her) has a Master's degree in Public Health with a focus on community health education and is a proud CHES®. After implementing and evaluating a successful flu campaign at her worksite, the local health department has asked her to join a community health coalition with the goal of increasing flu vaccinations among adults in the community. The local health department data show that only 60% of adults ages 18–64 received the flu shot the previous year. People under the age of 18 and over the age of 65 have much higher rates. The coalition wants to use existing materials developed by the CDC because they do not have a large budget and also do not want to create materials if high-quality materials already exist.

In the fall of 2023, the CDC released a new health communication campaign for flu vaccine season, *Wild to Mild*, that was designed to:

> ...share key information with the public about how getting a flu vaccine can reduce your risk of flu and its potentially serious outcomes. The campaign focuses on encouraging flu vaccination among higher risk groups, especially pregnant people and children, given drops in vaccination uptake in those groups since the COVID-19 pandemic.
>
> *(CDC, 2023d, para. 1)*

CDC developed the campaign aimed at the population of people who do not think the vaccine prevents illness. The message of this campaign focuses on how the vaccine can help reduce the severity of the flu if you get the flu. To learn more about the campaign and review campaign materials, please visit https://www.cdc.gov/flu/spotlights/2023-2024/new-campaign-wild-to-mild.htm.

Aisha and the coalition are excited to use the campaign materials from the CDC because they are in a community that also has a zoo. The campaign uses images of animals typically in a zoo and the coalition believes that this campaign will resonate with the community. The CDC provides multiple print and electronic campaign materials to implement the campaign in any community with ready-to-use graphics, blog posts, and social media posts. To review the available graphics and resources, please visit https://www.cdc.gov/flu/resource-center/shareable-resources.htm.

The coalition plans to evaluate the campaign next year to assess if the number of adults who received the flu vaccine in their community increased. Aisha will lead the evaluation efforts and present the comparison date to the coalition.

Summary

- There are many health communication channels to disseminate health campaigns. These can include mass media channels (television, videos, billboards, and radio), small media channels (brochures, fact sheets, infographics, and posters), and social media channels (Instagram and Facebook). Small and large group sessions are an additional channel HES can use to disseminate health information.
- Cultural competence and health literacy are essential components in all health communication strategies. These ensure that health communication messages are culturally appropriate and developed at an appropriate reading level using clear language. There are many tools and guides to aid HES in developing materials that include these components.
- There are health communication strategies that allow HES to customize messages based on the target audience. These include audience segmentation, tailoring, and refining messages. When messages are created using these strategies, they will be more effective in achieving the desired healthy behavior changes.

- HES need excellent oral and written communication skills to be successful in their careers. This includes being able to communicate effectively with colleagues, elected officials, and community partners. This can include delivering presentations, drafting community-wide emails, developing fact sheets, sharing talking points, and writing project reports and grants. Effective communication skills by HES can aid greatly in achieving successful outcomes.

Web Resources

- **CDC Health Communication Gateway**
  https://www.cdc.gov/healthcommunication/index.html
  This CDC website is a comprehensive resource for HES to develop effective health communication campaigns and more. The website includes websites, fact sheets, social media content, health campaign information, and toolkits.
- **CDC Health Communication Playbook**
  https://www.cdc.gov/nceh/clearwriting/docs/health-comm-playbook-508.pdf
  This CDC resource provides communication strategies for creating health messages for consumers and the media.
- **CDC Health Equity Guiding Principles for Inclusive Communication**
  https://www.cdc.gov/healthcommunication/HealthEquityGuidingPrinciples.pdf
  This is a two-page document from CDC provides guidance on incorporating health equity in health communication messages and campaigns.

References

Adgate, B. (2023). *Nielsen: AM/FM Radio Reaches 91% Of U.S. Adults Each Month.* https://www.forbes.com/sites/bradadgate/2023/07/26/nielsen-amfm-radio-reaches-91-of-us-adults-each-month/?sh=58cda3caa155

Allen, J.D., Fu, Q., Shrestha, S., Nguyen, K.H., Stopka, T.J., Cuevas, A., Corlin, L. (2022). Medical mistrust, discrimination, and COVID-19 vaccine behaviors among a national sample U.S. adults. *SSM Popul Health, 20*, 101278. https://doi.org/10.1016/j.ssmph

Bakerjian, D. (2023). Agency for healthcare quality and research. *Personal Health Literacy.* https://psnet.ahrq.gov/primer/personal-health-literacy#:~:text=Written%20materials%20should%20be%20at,already%20developed%20patient%20education%20materials

Centers for Disease Control and Prevention. (2018). *Crisis and Emergency Risk Communication.* https://emergency.cdc.gov/cerc/

Centers for Disease Control and Prevention. (2022a). *About the Campaign.* https://www.cdc.gov/hearher/about-the-campaign/index.html

Centers for Disease Control and Prevention. (2022b). *Culture and Language.* https://www.cdc.gov/healthliteracy/culture.html

Centers for Disease Control and Prevention. (2023a). *Burden of Cigarette Use in the U.S.* https://www.cdc.gov/tobacco/campaign/tips/resources/data/cigarette-smoking-in-united-states.html?s_cid=OSH_tips_GL0005&utm_source=google&utm_medium=cpc&utm_campaign=TipsRegular+2021%3BS%3BWL%3BBR%3BIMM%3BDTC%3BCO&utm_content=Smoking+-+Facts_E&utm_term=smoking+facts+and+statistics&gclid=Cj0KCQjw4vKpBhCZARIsAOKHoWSzwAqlDxFSuakQsL_0ooYMQvgd2ZyqsQE_Bj05uVHzXvXEU-M_Mn0aAhnrEALw_wcB&gclsrc=aw.ds#age_group

Centers for Disease Control and Prevention. (2023b). *Campaign Resources.* https://www.cdc.gov/tobacco/campaign/tips/resources/index.html

Centers for Disease Control and Prevention. (2023c). *Health Equity Guiding Principles for Inclusive Communication.* https://www.cdc.gov/healthcommunication/Health_Equity.html

Centers for Disease Control and Prevention. (2023d). *New Wild to Mild Campaign Drives Key Message to Tame Flu and Reset Expectations.* https://www.cdc.gov/flu/spotlights/2023-2024/new-campaign-wild-to-mild.htm

Communications Strategy Group. (2023). *The Importance of Health Awareness Campaigns.* https://wearecsg.com/blog/importance-of-health-awareness-campaigns/

Guide to Community Preventive Services. (2010). *Health Communication and Social Marketing: Campaigns that Include Mass Media and Health-Related Product Distribution.* https://www.thecommunityguide.org/findings/health-communication-and-social-marketing-campaigns-include-mass-media-and-health-related

Guide to Community Preventive Services. (2022). *New Publications Show Health Communication Works.* https://www.thecommunityguide.org/news/new-publications-show-health-communication-works.html

Murphy-Hoefer R., Davis K.C., King, B.A., Beistle, D., Rodes, R., & Graffunder, C. (2020). Association between the *Tips From Former Smokers* campaign and smoking cessation among adults, United States, 2012–2018. *Preventing Chronic Disease, 17,* 200052. https://doi.org/10.5888/pcd17.200052

National Commission for Health and Education Credentialing, Inc. (2020). *Areas of Responsibility, Competencies and Sub-competencies for Health Education Specialist Practice Analysis II 2020 (HESPA II 2020).* https://assets.speakcdn.com/assets/2251/hespa_competencies_and_sub-competencies_052020.pdf

Naegle, K.M. (2021). Ten simple rules for effective presentation slides. *PLoS Computational Biology, 17*(12), e1009554. https://doi.org/10.1371/journal.pcbi.1009554. https://www.ncbi.nlm.nih.gov/pmc/articles/PMC8638955/

Pew Research Center. (2021). *Social Media Use in 2021.* https://www.pewresearch.org/internet/2021/04/07/social-media-use-in-2021/

TvScientific. (2023). *The Big List of TV Viewership Statistics [Updated for 2023].* https://www.tvscientific.com/insight/tv-viewership-statistics

U.S. Department of Education. (2017). *National Center for Education Statistics, Program for the International Assessment of Adult Competencies (PIAAC), U.S. PIAAC 2017, U.S. PIAAC 2012/2014.* https://nces.ed.gov/fastfacts/display.asp?id=69

U.S. Department of Health and Human Services. (2010). *National Action Plan to Improve Health Literacy.* https://health.gov/our-work/national-health-initiatives/health-literacy/national-action-plan-improve-health-literacy

CHAPTER 8

Leading and Managing:
A Role for Everyone

Learning Objectives

After reading this chapter, learners will be able to:

- **Describe key leadership and management skills needed in the health education and promotion field**
- **Summarize principles for working successfully with individuals and groups**
- **List the types of tools available for leading teams and projects**
- **List a variety of job titles and opportunities that HES are qualified for**

Keywords

- Agenda
- Change Management
- Icebreakers
- Leadership
- Management
- Meeting Facilitation
- Mentor
- Project Management
- Performance Review
- Strategic Planning
- Supervision

Self-Reflection Question

Take a moment and reflect on these questions:

1. Describe the qualities of a leader whom you admire.
2. What are strategies for effective leadership when managing a project?
3. Is conflict avoidable on a team? Defend your response.

DOI: 10.4324/9781003504320-8

There is no one clear definition of what defines a leader or a manager. **Leadership** and **management** are often used interchangeably, but they are distinct descriptors. Nayar explains that leadership "refers to an individual's ability to influence, motivate, and enable others to contribute toward organizational success," while management "consists of controlling a group or a set of entities to accomplish a goal" (2013, para. 7). Effective leaders focus on developing team members with skills and inspire them in their roles, while managers typically ensure projects are on track and within budget (Taplin, 2023). Gray argues that "leaders shape culture and managers work within it" (2009, p. 208). In addition, the higher the number of individuals that HES can influence in their role, the higher the likelihood that they are a leader (Nayar, 2013). Czabanowska (2014) argues that "developing effective leadership is essential" and that it should happen "at every level" (p. 28). To be an effective HES and public health professional, it is necessary to have strong leadership and management skills at every level. This chapter will focus on the skills necessary for HES to lead and manage teams and work.

Eight Areas of Responsibility for CHES® and MCHES®

Effectively choosing, delivering, and evaluating health communication messages aligns with the following Area of Responsibility for CHES® and MCHES®.

Area VII: Leadership and Management

This area includes five competencies and 31 sub-competencies for creating effective health communication messaging (National Commission for Health and Education Credentialing, Inc. [NCHEC], 2020). This includes identifying, cultivating, and maintaining relationships with collaborating partners and interested parties; recruiting, hiring and training staff and volunteers; tracking expenses and ensuring projects stay within budgets; and, leading efforts to address systems level approaches to addressing complex health topics with diverse partners (NCHEC, 2020).

To learn more about the Areas of Responsibility, please visit https://www.nchec.org.

Qualities for Effective Leadership and Management

There are many qualities that can be identified for HES to be effective leaders and managers. Although the list of qualities and characteristics of effective leaders and managers can seem never-ending, there are several themes that emerge, as indicated in Table 8.1. HES and other public health professionals "should be driven by values of social justice, equity, honesty and responsibility, coupled with expertise, ability to discern trends in the midst of complexity and to capitalise on those trends by creating smart, adaptive strategies in an evolving environment" (Czabanowska, 2014, p. 30) In addition, they can make data-informed decisions and be transparent in sharing appropriate information. Finally, they are able to influence others, have the courage to take steps that may be unfamiliar or new, and offer hope. HES may not take on these types of responsibilities early in their careers, it is a likely progression over time.

HES with a CHES® or MCHES® certification must commit to performing their duties ethically. However, this expectation goes beyond the requirements to maintain

Table 8.1 Selection of Characteristics of Effective Leaders and Managers

Characteristics of Effective Leaders and Managers

Commitment to social justice, ethics, and trustworthiness	Ability to analyze complex information and identity priorities	Ability to influence others
Expert in the practice of public health	Ability to make data informed decisions	Courage to take steps that may be unfamiliar and new
Expert in relevant health topics	Ability to be transparent and provide appropriate information to others	Offer hope

a certification that not all HES acquire. The very foundation of the work of HES is to advance social justice, addressing and eliminating disparities, and seeking health equity. This requires that HES operate in a transparent and honest way to conduct their work. Trust is one of the most important qualities that HES have. Without trust, the content that health education and promotion professionals develop and the interventions and programs they lead will crumble. Being a leader requires the knowledge to share information with others that is appropriate to the situation. Certainly there may be times when HES cannot disclose information due to confidentiality requirements. At times, simply sharing that some information cannot be disclosed due to these requirements can be reassuring and aid in building and maintaining trust with others. HES are expected to develop their expertise to be a resource to their organization, community, and the field of public health. This can and must happen at every level of responsibility. Whether HES are early, mid, or advanced level they need to develop their expertise and then practice within the scope of that expertise, knowing when to defer to someone else who is more senior within the organization. Leaders and managers must be able to review various types of data from multiple sources and be able to identify trends, synthesize the information into digestible information for a variety of interested parties, and be able to identify prioritized needs. They must also be able to influence others, whether that is to convince others to join in on a project, change policy, fund a project, or to become a messenger on a shared new vision for health with others. According to Yphantides et al. (2015),

> Influence is essential to achieve wide-spread change. Ideally, it is grounded in knowledge, which can be gained through formal education and expertise, gained through involvement with a broad range of people and institutions, and based upon accomplishments that have brought recognition and respect.
>
> *(para. 12)*

Varma et al. (2021) argue that what public health professionals, including HES, need to also have "...is the boldness to make the big asks..." (para. 14) because "...many public health personnel learn to think only in terms of what's immediately feasible given current resources" (para. 16). Thinking creatively, strategically, and logically are all necessary for HES and public health professionals to achieve the goal of improved health outcomes for all. Finally, even in the face of real danger and lack of information, HES need to be providers of hope. Even during the early days of the COVID-19 pandemic, when information was scarce, those who work in infectious disease taught the world how to protect themselves with the knowledge that was available on disease transmission. According to Coughlin (2006),

> SIDEBAR: DID YOU KNOW?
>
> Effective leaders and managers recognize the value of learning from others. The Rural Health Information Hub hosts a podcast to provide rural health leaders and subject matter experts the opportunity to share "solutions to help meet rural communities' needs" (The Rural Health Information Hub, 2023, para. 1).
>
> To learn more about the podcast, please visit https://www.ruralhealth-info.org/podcast.

> Sustaining or fostering hope among people and communities is consistent with the virtuous conduct of public health. In the presence of natural and manmade disasters and socioeconomic, ecological, and public health challenges, hope can be a mediator of coping, recovery, and resilience.
>
> *(para. 5)*

The qualities of a leader align with the basic expectations of HES at every level. There is a role for every HES to lead and manage whether through everyday health challenges, chronic health issues, or in response to a pandemic.

Activity 8.1: Discussion

Take a moment and consider your thoughts on the following questions:

1. What are qualities of an effective supervisor?
2. Do you think is the difference in supervising volunteers versus staff members? If so, describe the differences.
3. What do you think is the hardest part about supervising a team? Why?

Skills for Leading Teams

There are many key skills necessary to lead teams effectively. This can include **supervision**, completing **performance reviews**, team building, supporting team members, and relationship building with community members.

Skills in Leading Teams and Managing Projects

There are a wide variety of skills necessary to effectively lead teams and manage projects. This chapter explores just a few of these.

Supervision

It is common practice for HES to supervise staff and volunteers in their role as a leader. Supervision can include several key responsibilities such as interviewing, hiring and selecting staff and volunteers, onboarding them to the organization and/or department, training them for their role, and providing guidance and supervision to them as they embark on their role. If a HES is able to be the one to select and hire staff and volunteers, then they may be more familiar with the work experience that new hire brings to their role. Onboarding is generally a prescribed process through an organization or agency and must be completed within a specified time period. This typically includes how to navigate internal technology and systems, such as how to access the network, set up an email account, and forward phone calls correctly. Training of staff and volunteers will vary by position, agency, and organization need. It will also vary depending on the existing skills that the staff or volunteer brings to the role. It is not uncommon for a HES to identify and develop a training plan for their staff as they are the experts in the role and can best prepare others to execute it effectively.

Activity 8.2: Practice your Skills

Suppose that you are the program director for a health education and promotion unit at a large worksite. The unit was developed after the company's leadership realized the impact of COVID-19 on the workforce. You were hired to primarily address stress, nutrition, and general well-being of employees. You have worked alone for the past two years to develop programs and drafting policies that support over 1,200 employees. These employees work hybrid work schedules across four locations in the city. You recently applied for and then received a grant to develop programs to support employees who are parents with children under the age of 12. The grant deliverables included a needs assessment, drafting a policy to support parents, and two programs or services. Write a job description for a HES to join your team using the following prompts:

- What is the main purpose of the HES position?
- What skills do you think the HES needs to be successful?
- How will you evaluate the success of the HES in the role?

Supervisors may need to create schedules for staff and volunteers. This may require that they assess staffing throughout the day or week and make adjustments to future schedules. It might also include forecasting staffing needs for large events without prior experience for staffing the event because it is new for the team. Supervisors also process time cards and monitor hours for staff and volunteers. Typically this is done because there is a budget associated with payroll for paid staff. Volunteers may need to track their time to report to another entity. For example, volunteers may be students who need to report a specific number of hours to comply with class requirements or service hours to graduate. This task of supervision can be incredibly time consuming and it is helpful to have a tracking mechanism in place that automates some of this work. Supervisors may have to sign off on completed time cards, including reviewing them for accuracy. Errors on time cards can cause a lot of issues if not addressed right away.

Paid staff may receive a paycheck for an incorrect amount and volunteers may not meet their requirements.

Supervisors typically attend organizational meetings and are expected to share information with their staff and volunteers on key policies, practices, and events that may impact them in their role. This may require regular one on one meetings with staff and volunteers and regular team meetings. This depends on the size of the team, the amount of information to share, the impact of the information on the team, and the preference of the supervisor.

Performance Reviews

Most organizations require an annual evaluation of work performed by employees. This evaluation is typically referred to as a performance review. This review is a summary of all the accomplishments over the performance period and a chance to identify opportunities for improvement. It is an opportunity for the supervisor and staff member to review what is going well and what are areas for improvement or professional growth. Having an area for improvement does not mean that an individual is performing poorly; rather, it can be an opportunity to identify opportunities for growth within the role and in consideration of future roles. For example, if a staff or volunteer is in an entry-level role in health communications, then seeking out additional training on utilizing new technology may be a benefit for the current role and a requirement for a promotion. Supervisors have an opportunity to inspire staff and volunteers with performance reviews and help them in their professional journey.

Performance reviews are typically prepared in a template that is used across the organization. Many organizations require staff, and sometimes volunteers, to complete a self-assessment of their performance before receiving feedback from their supervisor. The supervisor can use the information from the self-assessment to comment on areas where the staff member or volunteer have met or not met expectations. A self-evaluation may provide clarity for not meeting expectations, such as internal delays beyond the control of the staff or volunteer. Since the performance review process typically covers between ten and 12 months of work, it is strongly recommended that staff, volunteers, and supervisors maintain a log of work completed to make recalling information easier. Although completing a performance review may be tedious, it is a valuable process for staff and volunteers. Ultimately, performance reviews are a valuable tool in documenting the growth of staff and volunteers in their roles and an opportunity for supervisors to reflect on their supervision style as they support staff and volunteers in their professional journeys.

SIDEBAR: DID YOU KNOW?

There are many tools and guides to support supervisors. The Society for Human Resource Management is a member-based organization primarily for professionals who work in the area of human resources, hiring, training, discipline, and supervision. The organization offers free tools and publishes articles on common challenges that supervisors may need to respond to and address.

To learn more about the employee relations resources available from SHRM, please visit https://www.shrm.org/ResourcesAndTools/hr-topics/employee-relations.

Team Building

In addition to one on one supervision, leading staff and volunteers frequently includes team building. Whether a team is composed of three individuals or 100, team building refers to identifying opportunities to create and foster a culture of trust among the staff and volunteers who work together. Team building does not mean that staff and volunteers need to be friends; rather, it describes developing a culture of shared respect and commitment to the work. A positive team culture is necessary for successful collaboration and support. A strong team culture will ensure that team members know how to identify and offer ways to support one another professionally. For example, a team built on mutual respect and support will flourish when a new project is in development and roles are identified. Staff and volunteers may be able to offer their skills in a proactive way and step in to support one another when someone needs to stay away from the project. One team member stepping away would not be seen as a threat to the work being completed, rather an opportunity for others to step up and ensure that the desired outcomes are achieved together with the resources and capacity that is available.

Team building is an on-going process that requires intentionality. Typically, **icebreakers** are used for staff and volunteers to get to know each other through low-risk activities. The risk is low in terms of the amount of personal or professional disclosure and emotional vulnerability needed. Icebreakers can include sharing brief introductions and fun facts.

Activity 8.3: Practice your Skills

There are many kinds of icebreakers to help get to know each other and build trust. A simple internet search for the term *icebreaker* results in over 50 million websites with ideas. The key is to find something that you feel comfortable leading and processing with a team.

Conduct a brief search for an icebreaker activity and lead it in a small group. Then ask for feedback on the following:

- Did you explain the point of the icebreaker?
- Were your instructions clear?
- Did you have all the necessary supplies?
- Were you able to solicit participation by most individuals?

Based on the feedback that you receive, would you change the way that you facilitate the icebreaker in the future? If so, how?

Supporting Team Members

In addition to creating a culture of respect and support for a team, HES who are leading teams need to be able to support the mental health of staff and volunteers. The work of health education and promotion professionals is not easy. It can be emotionally taxing and can be met with resistance from policy makers, community members, and funders. Often, the work addresses chronic health conditions that require intentional efforts over a long period of time to even reap incremental improvements. Some health education and promotion professionals may be working in content areas

SIDEBAR: DID YOU KNOW?

To support HES and other public health leaders, CDC offers a free online training called *Understanding and Preventing Burnout among Public Health Workers: Guidance for Public Health Leaders*. This 3.5-hour training helps HES supervisors learn "strategies to prioritize employee health and well-being and prevent burnout" (CDC, 2023b, para. 3). To learn more about the training, please visit https://www.cdc.gov/niosh/learning/publichealthburnoutprevention/default.html.

The NACCHO also promotes several training tools for health education and promotion leaders to support staff and volunteers in a Public Health Workforce Resilience Resource Library. To access this library and explore the resources, please visit https://www.naccho.org/programs/our-covid-19-response/public-health-resilience.

that are challenging, like sex education, discrimination, poverty, and violence. This means that supervisors need to be trained on the signs and symptoms of stress and trauma in the workplace and be familiar with the resources available for staff and volunteers. It also means normalizing conversations about mental health and supporting self-care activities. This can be incorporated into team meetings and encouraged with flex-time schedules, especially when working irregular hours to attend and lead evening and weekend community events and programs. The Centers for Disease Control and Prevention (CDC) highlights that "... individual-level solutions like self-care and resilience training can help, [but] changing workplace policies and practices [is] the best way to address burnout" (2023a, para. 5). Depending on the organization that HES are employed in, it may mean that they are the best resource to help in identifying opportunities for improvement in workplace policies and practices that help to protect their staff.

Relationships with Community Members

Because of the nature of the work that HES do, they are often called upon to reach out to, engage, and convene community partners. Koh (2009) highlights that "[p]ublic health leaders must begin by acknowledging the extraordinary challenges of the discipline, not the least of which is the field's enormity of scope and goals" (p. S12). Koh further explains that "public health strives for the most lofty of aspirations" with goals such as addressing and eliminating health inequities to ensure overall well-being for all (2009, p. S12). Even more prominent is that HES leaders will work in communities with

> ...seemingly limitless numbers of stakeholders. The field encompasses a growing multiplicity of actors, representing a dizzying array of values and perspectives about ends, means, and responsibility. Today, a "typical" public health meeting may feature doctors, nurses, occupational therapists, social workers, government officials, business leaders, advocates, payers, providers, researchers, media experts, sanitarians, and, of course, concerned members of the lay public. After 9/11, such meetings are also more likely to include police, fire, and emergency

medical services personnel. This diversity of perspectives and values creates, on one hand, a rich, uncommon culture that links professionals from diverse backgrounds…

(Koh, 2009, p.S12)

This requires HES leaders to build relationships with individuals based on trust, respect, and effective communication. It also means that HES leaders need to be able to work with multiple interested parties on not just responding to a current crisis, but to identify sustainable and scale-able solutions. This takes time and may test the patience of everyone involved. HES leaders need to not only motivate continued action and support but also be an anchor when the efforts may be stalled or seem like they will not get the needed support to even get noticed. This may require a change in the culture of the community or system (Gray, 2009). Finally, HES and other public health "…leaders need to be enablers and facilitators who support groups in creating and achieving shared goals. This principle of leadership is reflected in the notion of empowerment that is central to health promotion: enabling people to improve their health and address its determinants" (Czabanowska, 2014, p. 30).

Skills for Managing Work

There are many key skills necessary to manage work effectively. These can include **strategic planning, project management, change management,** and **meeting facilitation**. These skills require additional skills in time management, organization, and effective verbal and written communication.

Strategic Planning

The Public Health Accreditation Board defined a strategic plan as a document that identifies what the organization wants to accomplish, the required action steps, the timeline for completing the action steps, and the evaluation process (2013). Strategic planning is a key component of planning and implementing public health interventions and programs. This includes identifying goals and objectives; using work plan templates; and, creating a robust evaluation plan to determine if the objectives were met. HES will use these skills and also collaborate across organizations to ensure that efforts are not duplicated or conflict with other projects.

> **SIDEBAR: DID YOU KNOW?**
>
> There are many leadership skills necessary to be an effective leader. Mind Tools offers a brief assessment tool to help you determine how good your own leadership skills are. To learn more, please visit https://www.mindtools.com/apdfhaw/how-good-are-your-leadership-skills.

> **SIDEBAR: DID YOU KNOW?**
>
> The National Association of County and City Health Officials (NACCHO) offers guides, workbooks, and examples of strategic plans on their website to help HES who are managing projects and leading teams.
>
> To review the available resources, please visit https://www.naccho.org/programs/public-health-infrastructure/performance-improvement/strategic-planning.

SIDEBAR: DID YOU KNOW?

The PMI offers multiple certifications in project management. This is a credential to recognize professionals with skills in planning, implementing, monitoring, and evaluating projects. A popular certification in the workplace is the Project Management Professional or PMP®. Prior to taking the exam, learners must complete a series of courses to learn specific frameworks and tools used in project management.

To learn more about the PMP® certification, please visit https://www.naccho.org/programs/public-health-infrastructure/performance-improvement/strategic-planning.

Project Management

Often, the work of HES involves managing a project. The Project Management Institute (PMI) defines project management as "...the use of specific knowledge, skills, tools and techniques to deliver something of value to people" (2023, para. 1). The projects include staff, budgets, and expected deliverables within a specific time frame (Project Management Institute, 2023). Basically, project management describes the skills HES use in managing the implementation and evaluation of interventions and programs. Beyond the health education and promotion field, these are invaluable skills to offer an employer.

Change Management

It is expected that HES leaders and managers will be supporting communities, workplaces, and organizations through some type of change. The premise of the health education and promotion field rests on the concept of behavior change, whether increasing or decreasing actions or behaviors that lead to increases or decreases in specific health outcomes. This can be done through individual, group, organization, and society level changes in knowledge, behavior, attitudes, and policies. Therefore, HES who are managing projects that lead to changes are engaging in change management. Miller (2020) describes change management as "...the process of guiding organizational change to fruition, from the earliest stages of conception and preparation, through implementation and, finally, to resolution" (para. 7). Managing a change process requires asking key questions (Miller, 2020), such as:

- What has happened that has led to a change being necessary?
- What is the plan to make the change possible?
- What is the plan for communicating the need for the change, the actions involved in the change, and how the change will impact individuals and the organization?
- What are the potential challenges for implementing the change and how can they be overcome?

Asking these questions can help the HES who are leading the project be better prepared in their role. However, the reality is that change can be unpredictable even with the best of planning. Things may not go as planned, reactions to the change(s) may fluctuate through the implementation process, and there may be additional factors impacting the need for a change that may not have been visible until the implementation process begins. Therefore, HES need to be able to pivot when needed and make adjustments as necessary while also maintaining open lines of communication with all who are involved and impacted.

Meeting Facilitation

HES and other public health professionals are often in roles that require them to facilitate meetings. Meetings are often necessary to bring interested parties together to brainstorm ideas and possible solutions before a project begins and throughout the life cycle of a project to address potential barriers and obstacles. Meetings are a way to share updates with others and explore next steps. Meetings can be short or long in length, varying from 15 minutes to multiple hours. The length of a meeting should be determined by the goal and purpose of the meeting.

> **SIDEBAR: DID YOU KNOW?**
>
> It is common for boards, commissions, and local government agencies to use Robert's Rules of Order to conduct meetings in an organized and logical manner (Robert's Rules Association, 2023). Using Robert's Rules of Order (Rules) in meetings may make them feel formal and rigid; however, the point of the Rules is to provide fair opportunities for all parties to speak and be heard in meetings. Some groups may choose to adopt only some of the Rules, while others will insist on using each of the Rules and have a presiding parliamentarian in place to ensure accuracy in use to discuss topics and conduct voting.
>
> To learn more about Robert's Rules of Order, please visit https://robertsrules.com/.

If the purpose of a meeting is clear, then it will guide what needs to be included in a meeting **agenda**. Meeting agendas are strongly recommended for every meeting. An agenda is a guiding document that outlines the plan for the meeting. Typical elements of an agenda include the date, location, and key items to cover. In the sample meeting agenda, indicated in Figure 8.1, the agenda can also include welcome traditions. In this agenda, the HES facilitating the meeting would provide an opportunity for meeting attendees to introduce themselves and welcome new members to the coalition. While the sample agenda only includes the total time dedicated for the meeting (from 4 to 5:30 pm), an agenda can designate a specific amount of time for each topic. For example, the welcome and introductions could be limited to ten minutes while the guest speaker may have 40 minutes. This type of addition to an agenda can help to keep the meeting on track to end in a timely manner. The sample agenda includes key topics such as an update from the Marketing and Policy committees and action items for each of them, such as a vote on a new logo design and soliciting feedback on the proposed changes to the policy. Agendas can also include key notes from prior meetings. The sample meeting agenda indicates the immediate and long-term needs of the coalition and these would be identified by the HES facilitating the meeting with input from any other project leadership. Another approach to building an agenda is to solicit ideas and suggestions at the end of one meeting for the subsequent meeting or communicate with the group prior to the next meeting to solicit ideas.

Coalition to End Drunk Driving
April 23, 2027 from 4 to 5:30 pm
Location: Annex Hall, Room 233 or Virtual using Zoom link

Welcome & Introductions

- Two new members RSVPed to attend today

Status update from Marketing Committee

- Vote on new logo design

Status update from Policy Committee

- Feedback on proposed policy changes

Guest Speaker: *Sabrina Holstead, CEO for Local Non-Profit*

Review of budget for upcoming awareness event

Need for volunteers for upcoming awareness event

Action items and next steps

Next meeting: May 23, 2027

Figure 8.1 Sample Meeting Agenda

Activity 8.4: Practice your Skills

Draft an agenda based on the following brief description of the objectives for an upcoming meeting of the project team you are leading using a template provided in Figure 8.1. The agenda should include time for each of the identified areas in the description in an order that is logical and timely. The meeting is typically scheduled to last one hour. You will need to determine if this meeting needs to last longer, and if so – how long should it last?

Meeting description: Last week, the project team members each shared an update on their work in preparation of the launch of the website as part of the new program. The group discovered a challenge with the tool where community members enter their zip code to locate the closest playground for children between the ages of 2 and 5. The system will not accept each of the seven zip codes in the city. In addition, leaders from the neighboring city want to collaborate and have their playgrounds included for an additional eight zip codes. The team needs to brainstorm how these issues will address the project timeline and impact the existing marketing efforts. In addition, a guest speaker from another city has agreed to come and share their successes and lessons learned with the project team.

Challenges in Leading and Managing

Chapter 10 explores the challenges and opportunities for today's public health workforce.

Leadership Development

There is a common belief that some people are born leaders. While that may seem true and accurately describe some individuals, the reality is that being an effective leader requires a commitment to ongoing professional development. According to Czabanowska (2014), "[p]rofessional development of public health leaders requires competency-based instruction to help them develop the abilities to address the complex and evolving demands of health care systems" (p. 29). Furthermore, Koh and Jacobson (2009) explain that:

> Aspiring public health leaders should not be left on their own to find guidance. Those with convening power can create new learning and teaching for the field by bringing together multiple parties, disseminating lessons learned from successful interventions and supporting those willing to take on the leadership challenge. Those who have successfully navigated these waters can share their insights as experienced change agents and coach those otherwise working in isolation, thereby providing another service in our service-oriented profession.
>
> *(para. 13)*

As such, there are many opportunities for HES at any level to learn, develop, and refine their leadership and management skills. This allows them to lead teams and ensure work deliverables are of high quality and completed within budget and in a timely manner. As indicated in Table 8.2, organizations such as the Public Health Foundation offer available training and resources on their website and through the TRAIN online learning platform (n.d.). The Public Health Institute Center for Health Leadership & Impact offers an application based program to work in multidisciplinary programs as part of a learning experience to address public health challenges within a community (2023).

Table 8.2 Organizations that Offer Leadership Development Training

Organization Name	Website	Description of Services
Public health foundation	https://www.phf.org/	Training and resources to support performance management, quality improvement, and workforce development[1]
Public health institute center for health leadership & impact	https://leadershipacademy.health/	A cohort based program where interdisciplinary teams of four are selected to address health issues in their community as part of an eight-month experience[2]
National network of public health institutes	https://www.phlearningnavigator.org/	This website offers curated asynchronous modules on topics such as leadership and best practices[3]

Note[1]: Adapted from "Focus Areas" by Public Health Foundation, n.d., Retrieved from https://www.phf.org/focusareas/Pages/default.aspx

Note[2]: Adapted from "Program overview" by Public Health Institute Center for Health Leadership & Impact, 2023, Important Dates, Cost & Funding. Retrieved from https://leadershipacademy.health/programs/overview/important-dates

Note[3]: Adapted from "Training search" by National Network of Public Health Institutes, 2023. Retrieved from https://www.phlearningnavigator.org/training/search

Professional Development

The next section identifies specific opportunities for leadership development. The topic of professional development for early, mid, and advanced level HES is the focus of Chapter 9.

Activity 8.5: Practice your Skills

Explore each of the resources provided in Table 8.2 and then select a free, one-hour course to complete from the National Network of Public Health Institutes (NNPHI).

1. What stands out to you about the resources available for developing leadership skills?
2. What course did you complete from the NNPHI? Why did you select that course?
3. Explain what you learned from the course you completed and why that is an important topic for HES leaders and managers to know.

According to the Canadian Public Health Association (CPHA), developing leadership skills can also happen through networking with other leaders in the field, finding a **mentor,** and asking for feedback whenever possible (2016). Identifying a public health leader that HES respect may be a helpful step. By doing this, HES may benefit by learning from others in public health that may have taken a professional pathway that is exciting and interesting to them. This could develop into a mentor/mentee relationship. Finally, the CPHA also recommends that HES interested in developing leadership skills take advantage of all opportunities to lead. The reality is that HES have these kinds of opportunities at every level. Though they may not encompass all the skills of an advanced-level leader, taking on these roles with the appropriate support and supervision can be an excellent opportunity to become a better leader in the future.

Job Roles and Opportunities

There are many job titles used to identify HES roles in the workplace and within communities. HES work in five primary settings, including public health departments, worksites, hospitals or healthcare organizations, nonprofits, and

SIDEBAR: DID YOU KNOW?

There are several popular job boards that post jobs in health education and promotion. These include, but are not limited to the following:

Public Health Employment Connection
Hosted by the Emory Rollins School of Public Health
Link: https://apps.sph.emory.edu/PHEC/

NCHEC Careers page
Hosted by the National Commission for Health Education Credentialing, Inc.
Link: https://www.nchec.org/job-postings

Idealist
Link: https://www.idealist.org/en

PublicHealthCareers.org
Managed by the Association of State and Territorial Health Officials
Link: https://www.publichealthcareers.org/

educational institutions (U.S. Bureau of Labor Statistics, 2022, What They Do, para. 4–8). A job title for HES working in community health education could include *community health educator* and *education program manager* (NCHEC, n.d.). In comparison, HES working in government or a local health department may have a job title as *health program analyst, advocate, or health information specialist.*

Common terminology used in early level job titles, as indicated in Table 8.3, include the terms *analyst* and *coordinator.* Typically the terms *lead* and *specialist* distinguish a mid-level HES, and *administrator* and *director* are associated with advanced level HES. Although these may be commonly used, they are not always used in the same way across agencies. For example, HES who lead health education and promotion programs may have a job title of *Health and Wellness Coordinator* or *Lead Health and Wellness Associate.* Job titles are also specific to an agency or organization and can vary between fields. For example, in the government sector, *analyst* may describe a mid to advanced level HES.

The most notable and accurate way to distinguish early, mid, and advanced level HES jobs is through a review of the job responsibilities. It is common for HES at each level to have administrative responsibilities to include report writing, presentations, and content development. Typically, mid and advanced level HES

have supervision and budget responsibilities in their job functions. However, at each level HES are expected to demonstrate leadership and management skills.

Table 8.3 Common Language in HES Job Titles

HES Level	Terms Used in Job Titles	
Early	Analyst	Coordinator
Mid	Lead	Specialist
Advanced	Administrator	Director

Concept in Action 8.1

Background: *Sam* (they/them) has worked at a local non-profit as a health programs coordinator for the past three years. They have a bachelor's degree in Health Education and Promotion. Sam's primary role is to develop educational content and health promotion programs for local communities within the region, with the support of a volunteer Board. *José* (he/his) has a master's in Public Health and directs chronic disease prevention at a local health department. He is a member of the volunteer Board for the local non-profit and has extensive experience supporting community programs.

Sam has been tasked with drafting a proposal for a community event to raise awareness about diabetes. Sam has worked on diabetes education programs in the past with José and is eager to present a proposal to the Board for approval. The proposal would include lessons learned from the previous events and recommendations for changes. For example, Sam and José learned that community members really liked having a physical activity component as part of the community event. They both agreed that adding in activities like jump rope competitions and yoga would generate a lot of interest.

Sam also really wants the event to be targeted just to Black women in the community, however over the past year the incidence of diabetes among men has steadily increased. Since Sam did not want to risk that the Board would reject the proposal to target only Black women, Sam decided to alter the stats for diabetes prevalence in the community to reflect a number higher than what was documented by the local health department.

José was aware that Sam was drafting the proposal and offered to help since he worked with Sam on this topic before. Sam declined the offer for help saying, "Thanks, but I think I have everything that I need." On the day of the presentation, Sam spoke about the previous community event and the lessons learned, without ever mentioning José and his contributions.

Activity 8.6: Discussion

After reviewing **Concept in Action 8.1**, consider these following questions:

1. What ethical dilemma did Sam initiate by altering the health statistics for the community?
2. Should Sam have mentioned José's work and contribution in the proposal? Why or why not?
3. How could the Board respond to the proposal if they discover the missing and inflated information?
4. If you were Sam's supervisor, how would you have responded to Sam's actions?
5. If you were José's supervisor, how would you have responded to Sam's actions?

Summary

■ Key skills necessary to lead teams effectively include supervision, completing performance reviews, team building, supporting team members, and supporting community members. Key skills to manage projects effectively include strategic planning, project management, change management, and meeting facilitation.

- Working successfully with diverse individuals and groups requires HES to intentionally build trust, be transparent, and use strong verbal and written communication skills.
- There are many free tools available to support HES who are leading teams and managing projects. These include webinars, resource guides, and leadership development programs.
- There are many job titles used to identify HES roles in the workplace and within communities. These can include terms such as analyst, coordinator, and specialist. To determine if the position is an early, mid, or advanced level, the job responsibilities in the position description need to be reviewed.

Web Resources

- **Video: Adaptive Leadership and Public Health**
  https://tinyurl.com/saewsze3
  NACCHO developed a 5 minute and 30 second video that explores the concept of adaptive leadership in public health.
- **Leadership Toolkit**
  https://publichealth.berkeley.edu/student-life/career-and-leadership-development/toolkit/
  The University of California, Berkeley School of Public Health offers a toolkit on leadership in public health on their website. The toolkit explores topics such as advocacy, career development, and self-care.
- **Video: 5 Steps in the Change Management Process**
  https://www.youtube.com/watch?v=wxVgd8h1svU
  Harvard Business School Online released this 3 minute and 30 second video on the five steps in the change management process as part of their Business: Explained video series.

References

Canadian Public Health Association. (2016). *Leadership in Public Health Practice* [PowerPoint Slides]. https://www.cpha.ca/sites/default/files/uploads/webinars/2016-09-14-vollman_public-health-leadership.pdf

Centers for Disease Control and Prevention. (2023a). *Support for Public Health Workers and Health Professionals.* https://www.cdc.gov/mentalhealth/public-health-workers/index.html

Centers for Disease Control and Prevention. (2023b). *Understanding and Preventing Burnout among Public Health Workers: Guidance for Public Health Leaders.* https://www.cdc.gov/niosh/learning/publichealthburnoutprevention/default.html

Coughlin, S.S. (2006). Hope, ethics, and public health. *Journal of Epidemiology and Community Health, 60*(10), 826–827. https://doi.org/10.1136/jech.2006.047431

Czabanowska, K. (2014). Leadership in public health: Reducing inequalities and improving health. *Eurohealth International, 20*(3), 28–31. https://iris.who.int/bitstream/handle/10665/332826/Eurohealth-20-3-28-31-eng.pdf?isAllowed=y&sequence=1

Gray, M. (2009). Public health leadership: creating the culture for the twenty-first century. *Journal of Public Health, 31*(2), 208–209. https://doi.org/10.1093/pubmed/fdp034

Koh, H.K. (2009). Leadership in public health. *Journal of Cancer Education, 24*(Suppl 2), S11–S18. https://doi.org/10.1007/BF03182303

Koh, H.K. & Jacobson, M. (2009). Fostering public health leadership. *Journal of Public Health,* *31*(2), 199–201. https://doi.org/10.1093/pubmed/fdp032

Miller, K. (2020). *5 Critical Steps in the Change Management Process.* https://online.hbs.edu/blog/post/change-management-process

National Commission for Health and Education Credentialing, Inc. (n.d.). *Guide to Health Education Careers.* https://www.nchec.org/guide-to-health-education-careers

National Commission for Health and Education Credentialing, Inc. (2020). *Areas of Responsibility, Competencies and Sub-competencies for Health Education Specialist Practice Analysis II 2020 (HESPA II 2020).* https://assets.speakcdn.com/assets/2251/hespa_competencies_and_sub-competencies_052020.pdf

National Network of Public Health Institutes. (2023). *Training Search.* https://www.phlearningnavigator.org/training/search

Nayar. V. (2013, August 2). *Three Differences between Managers and Leaders.* https://hbr.org/2013/08/tests-of-a-leadership-transiti

Project Management Institute. (2023). *What is Project Management?* https://www.pmi.org/about/learn-about-pmi/what-is-project-management

Public Health Accreditation Board. (2013). *Standards & Measures.* https://www.phaboard.org/wp-content/uploads/PHABSM_WEB_LR1.pdf

Public Health Foundation. (n.d.). *Focus Areas.* https://www.phf.org/focusareas/Pages/default.aspx

Public Health Institute Center for Health Leadership & Impact. (2023). *Program Overview.* https://leadershipacademy.health/programs/overview/important-dates

Robert's Rules Association. (2023). *Books.* https://robertsrules.com/books/

Taplin, S. (2023). *Manager versus Leader: What's the Difference?* https://www.forbes.com/sites/forbestechcouncil/2023/07/03/manager-versus-leader-whats-the-difference/?sh=714580e64540

The Rural Health Information Hub. (2023). *Exploring Rural Health Podcast.* https://www.ruralhealthinfo.org/podcast

U.S. Bureau of Labor Statistics. (2022, April 22). *Occupational Outlook Handbook, Health Education Specialists and Community Health Workers.* https://www.bls.gov/ooh/community-and-social-service/health-educators.htm

Varma, J.K., Long, T.G., & Chokshi, D. (2021). *5 Skills Public Health Officials Need to Combat the Next Pandemic.* https://hbr.org/2021/12/5-skills-public-health-officials-need-to-combat-the-next-pandemic

Yphantides, N., Escoboza, S., & Macchione, N. (2015). Leadership in public health: New competencies for the future. *Frontiers in Public Health,* *3*, 24. https://doi.org/10.3389/fpubh.2015.00024

CHAPTER 9

Professional Development: Strategies for Effectiveness

Learning Objectives

After reading this chapter, learners will be able to:

- Describe strategies for identifying and completing continuing professional development
- Identify opportunities to develop and refine skills through specialized certifications
- Explain the responsibility to contribute to the field of public health
- Compare how various professional organizations support HES

Keywords

- Asthma Educator Specialist (AE-C)
- Call for Proposals
- Certified Diabetes Care and Education Specialist®
- Certified in Public Health (CPH)

- Continuing Education
- Professional Development
- Professional Development Funds
- Professional Development Plan
- Subject Matter Expert (SME)

Self-Reflection Questions

Take a moment and reflect on these questions:

1. How can HES demonstrate that they are utilizing best practices and providing current and up to date content in health education and promotion efforts?
2. How can HES maintain their CHES® or MCHES® credentials?
3. What are ways that HES can contribute to the field of public health?

DOI: 10.4324/9781003504320-9

Continual learning, developing and refining skills, and contributing to the field of public health are important components of the health education and promotion profession. These activities are collectively known as **professional development**. This chapter will explain what is meant by professional development and how HES can access opportunities for early, mid, and advanced level skillbuilding to continue to learn new information and skills, refine their existing skill set, and contribute to the field of health education and promotion. For HES that are CHES® and MCHES®, maintaining these certifications requires intentionality and commitment for engaging in **continuing education** opportunities. Finally, the chapter will review some of the professional organizations that support HES in their professional development with various types of opportunities.

Continual Learning

Professional development refers to the process of "enhancing the knowledge, skills, and attitudes of health and education professionals so that they can more effectively implement strategies" (U.S. Department of Health and Human Services and Division of Adolescent and School Health, National Center for HIV/AIDS, Viral Hepatitis, STD, and TB Prevention, 2022, para. 2). Because health education and promotion activities are ultimately based on science, which is constantly evolving, professional development is a career-long endeavor. Experts use new knowledge and advances in science to update guidelines and recommendations for health consistently. As these are released, health education and promotion messages need to be updated. This is an example of why continually developing as a professional is necessary. Knowing that recommendations made ten years ago might not remain relevant today requires HES to stay informed. It is the responsibility of each HES to stay abreast of current science, evidence-based recommendations, and best practices in the field.

The importance of professional development is recognized and required in many other professional fields, particularly those that require certifications or evidence that the professional is completing continuing education requirements. There is a popular myth outside of these fields or among early career HES who are not certified with

---

SIDEBAR: DID YOU KNOW?

In 2008, the Physical Activity Guidelines for Americans were developed to serve as the "primary, authoritative voice of the federal government for evidence-based guidance on physical activity, fitness, and health for Americans" (U.S. Department of Health and Human Services and Office of Disease Prevention and Health Promotion [ODPHP], 2021, para. 2). In 2018, the second edition of the Physical Activity Guidelines for Americans, with recommendations for physical activity for individuals aged 3 and older, was released (ODPHP, 2021). To promote the guidelines the Move Your Way® campaign was developed with downloadable posters, videos, and factsheets about the specific recommendations with key messages for children, teens, and adults (ODPHP, 2023). These Guidelines are an example of changes and updates in health-related information that HES need to know.

To learn more about the specific recommendations, please visit https://health.gov/ and search for *Physical Activity Guidelines*.

CHES® and MCHES® credentials that professional development needs to occur only when an individual is well established in their career. In reality, professional development cannot be limited to advanced career professionals. Embracing this concept early is key to ensuring that ethical standards are maintained, current best practices are used in completing job responsibilities, and to support trust building with communities.

In addition, beyond completing a degree in health education and promotion or a related field, the recognition of professional development is an opportunity to consider what additional skills are needed for a HES to continue to advance in their career. Thinking about this early in a career can be quite exciting. HES may want to learn how to become a better educator and learn ways to incorporate principles for teaching youth and adults effectively. HES may recognize the value of networking, but are not sure how to network. HES may just want more opportunities to network. Finally, HES may seek out skills to better develop their leadership skills or their leadership style. Being intentional and thinking about an action plan like this can help HES grow professionally and potentially advance in their careers.

Many workplaces include the development of an action plan like this, typically referred to as a **professional development plan**, into employee performance reviews. This means that as part of goal setting for performance expectations on the job and an annual job evaluation, HES may be asked to identify what they want to pursue as part of their professional development plan. This plan may be reactive to an identified gap in skills that may have led to missed opportunities or a lower score on a performance evaluation. The plan could also be proactive allowing the HES to identify skills they want to develop or content that they want to learn.

Conferences and Workshops

Attending and participating in conferences and workshops are common ways for HES to learn about emerging health topics, research results, best practices, and resources. Conferences present information to attendees through plenary sessions that everyone attends, in breakout sessions, or a combination of both. Breakout sessions are smaller sessions that occur during a conference. Typically, multiple breakout sessions occur simultaneously on a variety of topics, and attendees select the session(s) that interest them the most. This means that they will have to miss some presentations. However, many conferences now make all of the speaker materials available at the conclusion of the conference so that attendees can review them despite not attending all sessions.

Conferences may also host poster sessions. These sessions are typically done in person with authors presenting a summary of information about research, interventions, or programs visually on a large poster. In response to COVID-19 and scheduled conferences during the lockdowns, remote versions of this type of session were developed. Some poster sessions may now include pre-recorded audio that can be reviewed by attendees asynchronously and on-demand on a virtual conference platform. Poster sessions offer conference attendees the opportunity to browse through various topics and content and ask questions of the presenter.

Conferences can range in length, from one day to a week, and occur in locations around the world. Typically conference organizers host conferences in different locations each year, sometimes with intentionality in hosting the conference in different

SIDEBAR: DID YOU KNOW?

Paying for professional development can add up. As a financial benefit to employees, employers may offer **professional development funds**. Professional development funds can be used to attend conferences and pay for the costs for obtaining and maintaining certifications. These funds can also be used for workshops, classes, and to complete an academic degree or certificate. Employees may be able to access these funds to pay for expenses directly or request a reimbursement from their employer.

Typically, this is a benefit that is included in a job description and discussed as part of the onboarding of new employees. If you have a job that has not offered professional development funds, it may be a good idea to inquire about it. Sometimes employers have this benefit and don't promote it well or they have not offered it to their workforce because they did not know that employees were interested.

parts of the state or country. Typically international organizations will rotate their conference to different host countries. The cost for attending a conference can vary from a few hundred to a few thousand dollars. Costs may include a registration fee for attending, travel costs, and costs of meals and lodging.

Not all conferences are held in person. The COVID pandemic forced many organizations to reconsider large gatherings and have found that virtual gatherings are more accessible and may increase their attendance. Many conferences can be quite successful and engaging when delivered virtually. Certainly the opportunities to connect with other students or professionals may be different, but virtual options are also typically less expensive and offer opportunities for participation for those that may not be able to afford the costs associated with travel and lodging for several days.

Literature

Another common strategy for HES to continually learn information on health topics or about best practices is by reviewing literature. This may include reading journals, like *Health Promotion Practice* and *The American Journal of Health Promotion*. This may also include reading newspaper publications such as *The Nation's Health* published by the American Public Health Association, known as APHA. These publications include research studies, editorial opinions, and information on current health topics. Depending on the nature of the study, the local or national media may promote the research findings, however, that does not always happen.

Although it is important for HES to maintain awareness of emerging evidence and science, this can be time-consuming and not always practical due to the volume of information that is available. One strategy HES can use to review summaries of key health research, current health issues, and changes in health recommendations is to sign up for organizational and departmental newsletters. Newsletters are typically released by non-profit organizations and various government agencies and departments to deliver this type of information to consumers and public health professionals. These newsletters are available free of charge, without any further obligations, and are delivered to email boxes on a regular basis. The number of issues may vary across organizations; however, it is common to receive a newsletter on a monthly basis.

Activity 9.1: Practice your Skills

Professional newsletters are available on a wide variety of topics. Finding newsletters to receive is actually quite easy. Simply follow these directions and find a newsletter that is of interest to you.

1. Search for *Public Health Newsletters* in your internet browser. Typically, search results include newsletters distributed by academic institutions, local and federal government departments and agencies, and public health organizations, such as the APHA.
2. Search for newsletters on specific public health issues by adding the topic to the search terms. For example, search for *Public Health Diabetes Newsletters* or *Public Health Advocacy Newsletters*. Multiple options will be available.

It may take a cycle before you receive a newsletter in your email inbox. When you do, be sure to review the newsletter for current topics. You may be surprised at the volume of information that is included and the kinds of opportunities listed. For example, newsletters may contain links for current job opportunities, professional development sessions, and more.

Current Events

Staying informed about current events is also a strategy for continual learning. Monitoring local, state, regional, and national news outlets can be a good way to stay informed about advances in health research and evidence-based recommendations. For HES who work primarily at the local level, knowing what the local news outlets are and accessing them regularly can offer valuable insight on emerging issues. For example, there may be a spike in crime in a specific part of a town and in response there may be community gatherings about how to react to and manage the situation. HES who are working to support the mental health of residents may consider participating in the event to offer information about available resources in the community to those who may be struggling. It is also important to be informed about global events as they can impact local communities in a wide variety of ways. There may be an increase in military deployments that may impact residents who are Service members. Residents who have family and friends abroad may need additional support processing events they are reading about and seeing on social media. There may be humanitarian responses, like food drives and fundraisers. The point is that HES really do need to know the community that they are working in and be informed about the concerns that matter to them. This will help HES build relationships with community members that are genuine and authentic.

Developing and Refining Skills

In addition to continual learning, developing and refining skills is another key component of professional development for HES. This can apply to early, mid and advanced HES. Developing and refining skills is about finding ways to further help a community. For example, suppose a HES was initially hired to develop a program on nutrition but then after a successful implementation realized that there was interest within the organization and community to focus next on physical activity. The HES may have a basic level of knowledge on the topic, but to better serve the needs of the organization and the community they want to become a yoga instructor and co-lead sessions.

When considering opportunities to develop and refine skills, HES may decide to specialize in a specific content area or skill set. This type of specialization is often referred to subject matter expertise and an individual with this level of knowledge and experience is referred to as a **Subject Matter Expert** or a SME. Typically, mid and advanced career HES are considered to be SMEs. After acquiring additional knowledge or mastering a skill set, HES may want to consider additional certifications. These are typically completed in addition to obtaining CHES® or MCHES® credentials. It is not uncommon to meet mid and advanced HES with several acronyms after their last name, specifying a number of certifications and credentials.

These additional credentials can include a **Certified in Public Health (CPH)** credential, a **Certified Diabetes Care and Education Specialist®** credential, and an **Asthma Educator Specialist (AE-C)**. HES can also specialize in skills that support system level strategies, such as policy development or grant writing. HES who have advanced skills in these areas are also considered SMEs.

Certified in Public Health

A popular and relevant voluntary national certification HES can acquire is the Certified in Public Health (CPH) credential, managed by the National Board of Public Health Examiners (NBPHE). In collaboration with the American Public Health Association, the Association of Prevention Teaching and Research, the Association of Schools and Programs of Public Health, the Association of State and Territorial Health Officials, and the National Association of County and City Health Officials, the NBPHE was founded in 2005 to " ...ensure that public health professionals have mastered the foundational knowledge and skills relevant to contemporary public health" (The National Board of Public Health Examiners [NBPHE], 2023a, para. 1).

From the late 1980s until 2005, multiple research efforts and meetings were conducted to determine the level of support and feasibility of a national certification in public health (NBPHE, 2023a, NBPHE History). The release of the first set of competencies for MPH graduates and the inaugural meeting of the NBPHE occurred in 2005 (NBPHE, 2023a, NBPHE History). By 2008, the first exam was offered and over 500 public health professionals were credentialed as Certified in Public Health (CPH) (NBPHE, 2023a, NBPHE History). By 2012, the exam was offered twice a year; by 2017, the exam was offered year-round at independent testing sites; and by 2020, the exam was available with live-proctoring (NBPHE, 2023a, NBPHE History). In 2014, a Job Task Analysis was performed, and in 2019, the exam was updated to meet the revised competencies and job functions (NBPHE, 2023a, NBPHE History).

Summary of CPH Domains

While the CHES® and MCHES® exam is based on eight Areas of Responsibility, the CPH exam is based on ten domains indicated in Table 9.1. The domains include Evidence-based Approaches to Public Health, Communication, Leadership, Law and Ethics, Public Health Biology and Human Disease Risk, Collaboration and Partnership,

Table 9.1 Ten CPH Domains

CPH Domains	
Evidence-based approaches to public health	Collaboration and partnership
Communication	Program planning and evaluation
Leadership	Program management
Law and Ethics	Policy in public health
Public health biology and human disease risk	Health equity and social justice

Note: Adapted from "CPH Exam Content Outline" by NBPHE, 2019, p. 1–4. Retrieved from https://nbphe-wp-production.s3.amazonaws.com/app/uploads/2017/05/ContentOutlineMay-21-2019.pdf

Program Planning and Evaluation, Program Management, Policy in Public Health, and Health Equity and Social Justice (NBPHE, 2023b). In the next section, each domain will be introduced with examples of how HES may demonstrate these in the workplace.

Evidence-based Approaches to Public Health. This domain examines how the practice of public health evolves; how research data is collected, analyzed, and interpreted; and how the process of reviewing data is under continuous review and improvement. It also includes the standardization of theories and models that are used to translate evidence-based approaches from research to practice.

Communication. To address health literacy and cultural competence needs, effective and timely communication of important health information is critical. This domain includes the practice of tailoring messages based on principles of health equity, identifying health disparities, and recognizing the communication needs of diverse groups.

Leadership. The COVID-19 pandemic has emphasized that leadership in public health at the organization level is critical for population health. The topics explored in this domain include workforce development, crisis management, stakeholder engagement, and quality assurance practices.

Law and Ethics. In an effort to focus on health equity and social justice, public health professionals must abide by ethical guidelines for public health professionals. This domain includes the practice of making informed decisions during training, research, program implementation, and other related activities by applying ethical considerations and guidelines.

Public Health Biology and Human Disease Risk. This domain explores studying risk factors for communicable and noncommunicable diseases on a continuous basis. This includes investigating the where, what, why, how, and when disease incidence and prevalence occur.

Collaboration and Partnership. Public health is everywhere and to be successful in achieving positive health outcomes, this domain explores how public health relies on the work and collaboration of many partners, including sectors such as transportation, housing, media, schools, worksites, government, faith-based organizations, and public safety. Public health is not the responsibility of one agency or organization, but rather a network or system of individuals and groups committed to improving health outcomes.

Program Planning and Evaluation. Health promotion program planning and evaluation must be integral components of the work that HES complete. This domain is about the practice of sharing lessons learned and best practices for continued development, evaluation and improvement of public health interventions.

Program Management. Managing programs, including personnel, budgets, work plans and timelines, is an important skill for HES to develop over time and included in this domain. These skills are critical for health promotion program implementation as the sustainability of these efforts depends on successful and resourceful leadership and management.

Policy in Public Health. Local, state, and federal policies can have meaningful and impactful outcomes and consequences for population health. This domain includes the impacts of ordinances, regulations, laws, legislation, and guidelines. These strategies can be influenced by elected officials and lobbyists. HES can provide valuable education on the impact of policies on health outcomes and serve as liaisons between community members and elected officials.

Health Equity and Social Justice. By using health equity and social justice lenses, HES can make a difference in the identification of and work to eliminate health disparities. This domain includes the application of various models to guide health promotion activities to address identified needs and gaps at multiple levels.

Eligibility Requirements

According to NBPHE (2023c), the following meet the eligibility requirements for the CPH exam:

- Current student of a school or program of public health accredited by the Council on Education for Public Health (CEPH);
- Alumni of a school or program of public health accredited by CEPH;
  - Individuals who have at least a bachelor's degree and at least five years' public health work experience;
  - Individuals with a relevant graduate-level degree and at least three years' public health work experience; or
  - Individuals with a graduate certificate from a school or program of public health that is accredited by or in applicant status with CEPH, and at least three years' public health work experience.

SIDEBAR: DID YOU KNOW?

CHES® and MCHES® are eligible for the **Asthma Educator Specialist (AE-C)** credential to signify their specialized knowledge of asthma and its impact on health (The National Board of Respiratory Care, 2023). To learn more about the eligibility requirements for obtaining AE-C credentials, please visithttps://www.nbrc.org/examinations/certified-asthma-educator-ae-c/.

MCHES® are eligible for the **Certified Diabetes Care and Education Specialist®** (**CDCES®**) credential if they also meet the additional requirements of professional practice experience and the number of hours they have documented of delivering diabetes care and education (Certification Board for Diabetes Care and Education, 2023, p. 8). To learn more about the eligibility requirements for obtaining CDCES® credentials, please visit https://www.cbdce.org/.

Test Format

The CPH exam consists of 200 questions, 175 of which are scored (NBPHE, 2021). The exam contains 20 questions from each of the ten domains (NBPHE, 2023b, para. 2). The test is timed and must be completed within four hours (NBPHE, 2021). NBPHE (2021) states that the pass rate is between 75% and 85% (p. 19).

Contributing to the Field of Public Health

HES are often in positions where they are able to glean valuable lessons and information from their work and HES have a responsibility to share this with others to contribute to the field overall. Lessons can range from best practices on how to do the work or about the interventions or programs that they implemented in their community. Perhaps the program evaluation revealed some key pieces about how to successfully implement the intervention in a rural community. This may be useful for HES working in rural communities to know, especially if all the examples about this particular program in the available literature highlight successful efforts only in urban settings. These types of articles about best practices and evaluation findings are typically submitted to a journal for peer review and publication.

There are many professional journals to consider. Some may be focused specifically on public health, health education and promotion, or just education. Once a journal has been identified the HES and any additional authors that will draft the manuscript will need to carefully review the submission guidelines. These guidelines will identify when manuscripts can be submitted as well as details about length, authorship, and format. Some journals will accept submissions throughout the year, while others may only accept submissions at specific times during the year and on limited topics. Manuscripts may be rejected simply for not complying with one or more of these criteria.

Once submitted, the journal editor assigns it to two to five volunteer reviewers. The article, often called a manuscript at this point, is then either accepted for publication or, as is often the case, sent back to the author(s) for revisions. The manuscript can also be rejected and the authors may want to consider identifying a different journal to submit the manuscript to.

Eight Areas of Responsibility for CHES® and MCHES®

Acting as an ethical professional and serving as a subject matter expert align with the following Area of Responsibility for CHES® and MCHES®:

Area VIII: Ethics and Professionalism

This Area includes four competencies and 21 sub-competencies that include maintaining ethical standards, promoting the health education and health promotion field and serving as a resource person and providing technical assistance to community groups (National Commission for Health and Education Credentialing, Inc. [NCHEC], 2020). This Area also incorporates professional development that CHES® and MCHES® are required to complete to stay up to date and current in their career (NCHEC, 2020).

To learn more about the Areas of Responsibility, please visit https://www.nchec.org.

Another avenue to share findings is to present at a local, state, regional, national or international conference. Typically there is a **call for proposals**. This is the official announcement requesting for those who wish to present to submit a proposal for acceptance. The announcement will include detailed instructions on the types of sessions that are available at the conference (plenary, breakout, poster) and the required information for a presentation to be considered. In most cases, proposals are reviewed by volunteer peers who are part of a committee to decide which proposals are accepted.

Depending on the conference, the organizers of the conference will develop an agenda of events in addition to the selected proposals. In this case, HES may be invited to give a presentation alone or as part of a panel. Some conferences also accept proposals for a panel presentation. This means HES can submit a proposal that identifies individuals that will be part of a panel and either provide prepared remarks and/or respond to audience questions. If a proposal is not selected for an oral presentation, it is relatively common that a poster presentation might be offered as an alternative option. Poster sessions offer a great opportunity for HES to meet and network with colleagues.

Concept in Action 9.1

Background: Sam (they/them) has worked at a local non-profit as a health programs coordinator for the past three years. They have a bachelor's degree in Health Education and Promotion. Sam's primary role is to develop educational content and health promotion programs for local communities within the region, with the support of a volunteer Board.

Sam is an active member of a state organization that brings together health education and promotion professionals on a yearly basis to network and share best practices. Recently, Sam collaborated with a local police and fire department to lead educational training sessions on opioids. The program was incredibly successful and the evaluation revealed other training topics that are of interest to the first responders. Sam noticed that there was a call for proposals for the conference next spring.

The call for proposals required the following elements for submissions:

1. Session Type (30-, 50-, or 90-minute session)
2. Session Title
3. Target Audience (Entry-, Mid- or Advance-level HES)
4. Abstract (limited to 50 words, describing content)
5. Three Learning Objectives

Sam has never submitted a conference proposal before but generally felt confident in being able to draft these items, except for the three learning objectives. Sam discussed the idea of submitting a conference proposal with their supervisor at a one on one meeting. Sam's supervisor was impressed that Sam was planning to submit a proposal and fully supported Sam in doing so. Sam's supervisor offered a graphic from Vanderbilt University to help guide Sam's development of the three learning objectives. The graphic (as indicated in Figure 9.1) explains Bloom's Taxonomy and provides examples for meaning learning objectives.

Based on this information, Sam developed the following learning objectives for the conference proposal:

By the end of the session, participants will be able to

- Duplicate the opioid program with police and departments
- Interpret evaluation feedback for training needs for first responders
- Design culturally responsive programs for first responders on key health topics

These three learning outcomes are aligned with Sam's proposed session abstract and use verbs from different levels of Bloom's Taxonomy to provide a meaningful learning experience and offer a training session that meets the needs of the conference attendees. Sam submitted the proposal and was accepted to present in the spring.

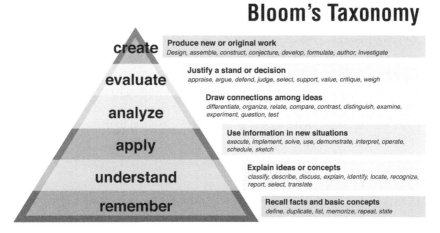

Figure 9.1 Bloom's Taxonomy

Note: From Vanderbilt University. (2023). Bloom's Taxonomy. Retrieved from https://cft.vanderbilt. edu/guides-sub-pages/blooms-taxonomy/#:~:text=Familiarly%20known%20as%20Bloom's%20 Taxonomy, Analysis%2C%20Synthesis%2C%20and%20Evaluation. Released under a Creative Commons Attribution license.

HES can also contribute to the knowledge base of the field by writing opinion articles, blog posts and related media, and books. HES are often asked to add content to their organization's website and post regularly on various social media platforms. For example, a local news organization might reach out to a HES for an interview on the current status of COVID-19 in the community. The interview might appear on TV, on the news organization's website and the HES might post it on their own LinkedIn profile as a way to share the news of a professional achievement and to further distribute the information on COVID-19.

SIDEBAR: DID YOU KNOW?

LinkedIn can also be a great tool for HES to network with other HES and public health professionals. A basic profile is available free of charge and provides an opportunity to describe the current job a HES has and information on their past work experience and key accomplishments. If you do not already have a LinkedIn profile, consider creating one – especially when you are job searching. It is also a great way to network.

To learn more about LinkedIn and to create a profile, please visit https://www. linkedin.com/.

Activity 9.2: Practice your Skills

Identify a HES in your community that you can either interview about their role or shadow for a few hours or a day. HES really appreciate students who reach out with an interest in learning more because there are so many different aspects to these roles that can be difficult to capture in an academic curriculum. In addition, HES also value networking, or connecting with other professionals with similar job responsibilities. Networking is also a good way to connect with potential partners, community members, and collaborators.

Once you have identified a HES, reach out and make your request. Once you complete the interview or shadow experience write a profile about their role and share it with your peers. Be sure to learn about their prior experience before being hired for their current role, describe key aspects of their current role, and share any observations you noticed such as job challenges and successes. Make sure to send a thank you email to the HES you shadowed.

Maintaining CHES and MCHES Credentials

An important part of being an ethical professional is maintaining earned credentials throughout one's career. An initial award of a credential will come with an expiration date. After this date, the credential may no longer be viable unless the HES demonstrates that they have engaged in approved activities to increase their knowledge and skill set. This involves completing continuing education contact hours. These continuing education contact hours are referred to as CECH for the CHES® and MCHES® credential and recertification credits for the CPH credential. There are many opportunities to complete tasks to earn these hours or credits and each certifying body has detailed information on the recertification process. They also curate a list of opportunities on their respective websites. This is generally true of other professions that require credentialing and the subsequent maintenance of those credentials.

CHES® and MCHES® are required to earn 75 CECH every five years (NCHEC, n.d.-a, n.d.-b). In addition, five of those 75 CECH must be Continuing Competency credits. Continuing Competency credits can be earned by taking a quiz following designated learning events or by providing an evaluation of job duties by a current supervisor (NCHEC, n.d.-a, n.d.-b). Of these CECH, 45 must come from providers who have been pre-approved to deliver continuing education, called Category 1 (NCHEC, n.d.-a, n.d.-b). The remaining CECH can be learning opportunities that are not pre-approved, called Category 2 (NCHEC, n.d.-a, n.d.-b). To receive credit for these, CHES® or MCHES® must document which of the Eight Areas of Responsibility and corresponding competences and sub-competencies (for MCHES®) the Category 2 CECH covered (NCHEC, n.d.-a, n.d.-b). In addition, some work functions can count as Category 2 activities. For example, giving a presentation, developing a curriculum, precepting an intern, and writing a successful grant application could all be counted.

SIDEBAR: DID YOU KNOW?

As part of the renewal process for CHES® and MCHES®, individuals are required to review the Code of Ethics for the Health Education Profession® and indicate that they have read and understood it and commit to practicing these standards.

To learn more about the Code of Ethics for the Health Education Profession® for CHES® and MCHES®, please visit https://www.nchec.org/code-of-ethics.

Professional Organizations

HES can benefit from ongoing mentorship and guidance from supervisors and public health professionals with significant work experience, especially after acquiring an entry level role in the field. As HES become more experienced themselves, they often find themselves serving as mentors to early career HES and as preceptors to students completing internships for health related majors and other academic programs. These relationships can often span decades and grow into personal friendships over time.

A great strategy for meeting other professionals and networking within the field is to join a professional organization. The benefits of these kinds of memberships include access to continuing education opportunities, current job postings, advocacy training and leadership opportunities. These types of organizations also offer scholarships to support attendance and participation at regional, state and national conferences.

Many of the organizations also publish peer-reviewed journals. Access to these can be included in membership dues. While there are many public health professional organizations that cater to one specific health topic, there are a few that broadly cover the field. Two of these are the American Public Health Association (APHA) and the Society for Public Health Education (SOPHE).

APHA

The APHA, founded in 1872, is the leading national professional organization for public health professionals with over 25,000 members from over 40 countries and governed by a 24-member board (American Public Health Association [APHA], 2023a). APHA supports the profession by championing the health of all people from all communities through advocacy, education, and focusing on health topics, issues, and policies that are supported by science. APHA is the publisher of the *American Journal of Public Health* and *The Nation's Health* newspaper (APHA, 2023a). These two highly regarded publications support HES and other public health professionals by providing timely and important information and research in the field.

Activity 9.3: Discussion

Visit APHA's website at https://www.apha.org/What-is-public-health and watch the 4-minute video, *What is Public Health* and respond to the following questions.

1. List of everything the video mentions is an example of public health.
2. Did anything in the video surprise you?
3. Did the video include anything that you had not thought of as a public health topic?

APHA offers professionals multiple opportunities to get involved. This includes attending and participating in the Annual Meeting and Expo and joining Special Primary Interest Groups. APHA supports the profession with social media, toolkits, fact sheets and more that are ready for use by HES in their roles. These are all readily available on their website at https://www.apha.org/.

Take a moment to review the website for current hot topics, upcoming conferences and events, job postings, press releases, publications, and continuing education opportunities. You may consider joining your state's public health association as a student to get a discounted membership. Students are eligible for discounted rates to attend conferences.

Activity 9.4: Discussion

Review the mission, vision, and values of the APHA posted on the APHA website:

APHA's Mission: "Improve the health of the public and achieve equity in health status" (APHA, 2023b, para. 2).

APHA's Vision: "Create the healthiest nation in one generation" (APHA, 2023b, para. 1; APHA, 2023d).

APHA's Values: Our values reflect the beliefs of our members from all disciplines of public health and over 40 countries: community, science, and evidence-based decision-making, health equity, prevention and wellness, real progress in improving health (APHA, 2023c).

Respond to the following questions and defend your response.

1. How can HES contribute to the mission and vision of the APHA?
2. Is achieving the healthiest nation in one generation possible?

For more information about APHA, please visit https://www.apha.org/About-APHA.

SOPHE

SOPHE is smaller than APHA and focuses specifically on health education and promotion professionals. Founded in 1950, it has members from around the world who work in a variety of settings, including schools, worksites, healthcare organizations, government agencies, and other nonprofit organizations (Society for Public Health Education [SOPHE], 2023). SOPHE supports the work of HES to include the promotion of health equity and healthy behaviors, communities and environments. SOPHE focuses on "... advanc[ing efforts] in health education theory and research, [promoting] excellence in professional preparation and practice, advocacy for public policies conducive to health, [and promoting] achievement of health equity for all" (SOPHE, 2023, para. 4).

Activity 9.5: Practice your Skills

Visit National SOPHE's website at https://www.sophe.org/membership/ and complete the following tasks:

1. Review the benefits of membership, including student membership.
2. Explore the website for upcoming conferences and events, job postings, press releases, and continuing education opportunities. Similar to APHA, students can join and attend conferences for a discounted membership.
3. Review the description of a Community of Practice (also referred to as a CoP) and identify which one(s) you may be interested in.
4. Determine if your state has a SOPHE chapter.

Other Specialized Professional Organizations

There are many other professional organizations that focus on a specific health topic, such as diabetes, cancer, lung health, aging, Alzheimer's disease, autism, and school health. As HES advance in their careers, they may join one or more of these

Table 9.2 Examples of Specialized Professional Organizations

Organization Name	Website
American Society on Aging	https://www.asaging.org/
American School Health Association	https://www.ashaweb.org/
National Association of Chronic Disease Directors	https://chronicdisease.org/
National Association of Diabetes Care and Education Specialists	https://www.diabeteseducator.org
Society of Health and Physical Educators	https://www.shapeamerica.org/
International Association of Providers of AIDS Care	https://www.iapac.org/

organizations particularly as they become specialists or subject matter experts in a health topic area. A few examples of these specialized professional organizations are provided in Table 9.2, including the American Society on Aging, the American School Health Association, the National Association of Chronic Disease Directors, the National Association of Diabetes Care and Education Specialists, the Society of Health and Physical Educators, and the International Association of Providers of AIDS Care.

These and other similar professional organizations and associations allow for HES and other colleagues to network, share information and collaborate on projects. These groups may convene state and national conferences, offer continuing education opportunities, and publish journals on their specific health topic.

Activity 9.6: Discussion
Review at least one of the specialized professional organizations listed in Table 9.2 and answer the following questions.

1. What is the organization's mission?
2. Is this a member organization? If so, who are the members?
3. In what ways does the organization support its members?

There are many other specialized professional organizations for HES. Simply search for *public health organization* and *any topic or role.* Review the list of results and select one organization website to review that is of interest to you. Then answer the following questions.

1. What is the organization's mission?
2. Is this a member organization? If so, who are the members?
3. How does the organization support its members?

Summary
■ Continual learning, developing and refining skills, and contributing to the field of public health are important components of the health education and promotion profession. Strategies for identifying and completing continuing professional development include attending and participating in conferences and workshops, reviewing relevant literature and being informed of current events. This can also include

- maintaining existing credentials and sharing knowledge, best practices, and other insights by presenting at conferences, publishing, and disseminating information through multiple channels, such as social media.
- After acquiring additional knowledge or mastering a skill set, HES may want to consider additional certifications. These are typically completed in addition to obtaining CHES® or MCHES® credentials. Specialized certifications can include Certified in Public Health (CPH), Certified Diabetes Care and Education Specialist®, and Asthma Educator Specialist (AE-C).
- HES can offer valuable insight to other HES and public health professionals based on the valuable lessons and information from their work. HES have a responsibility to share this with others to contribute to the field overall to advance best practices and contribute knowledge to the field. Lessons can range from best practices on how to do the work or about the interventions or programs that they implemented in their community.
- There are many professional organizations that HES can join during their careers. This includes APHA and SOPHE. These organizations provide many opportunities for HES to network, learn and share. HES can connect with others in the public health field from right in their own back yards to all over the world.

Web Resources

- **American Public Health Association (APHA)**
  https://www.apha.org/
  The American Public Health Association is a member organization that support public health professionals.
- **National Board of Public Health Examiners (NBPHE)**
  https://www.nbphe.org
  The National Board of Public Health Examiners administers the Certified in Public Health credential.
- **Society for Public Health Education (SOPHE)**
  https://www.sophe.org/
  The Society for Public Health Education is a member organization for health education and promotion professionals.
- **The Nation's Health**
  https://www.thenationshealth.org/
  The Nation's Health is a monthly newspaper publication by the American Public Health Association.
- **Comparison of CHES® and CPH**
  https://www.nchec.org/cph-and-ches
  This graphic developed by NCHEC compares the differences in eligibility, exam details, and other important information between the two certifications.

References

American Public Health Association. (2023a). *About APHA*. https://www.apha.org/About-APHA

American Public Health Association. (2023b). *Our Mission*. https://www.apha.org/About-APHA/Our-Mission

American Public Health Association. (2023c). *Our Values*. https://www.apha.org/About-APHA/Our-values

American Public Health Association. (2023d). *Our Vision*. https://www.apha.org/About-APHA/Our-Vision

Certification Board for Diabetes Care and Education. (2023). 2023 *Certification Examination for Diabetes Care and Education Specialists Handbook*. https://www.cbdce.org/documents/20123/66178/CBDCE-exam-handbook_Current.pdf/8e2fda09-9289-947c-7587-712a4e74f10a?t=1588269156519

National Board of Public Health Examiners. (2019). *CPH Exam Content Outline*. https://nbphe-wp-production.s3.amazonaws.com/app/uploads/2017/05/ContentOutlineMay-21-2019.pdf

National Board of Public Health Examiners. (2021). *CPH Candidate Handbook*. https://nbphe-wp-production.s3.amazonaws.com/app/uploads/2017/05/CPH-Candidate-HAndbook.pdf

National Board of Public Health Examiners. (2023a). *About NBPHE*. https://www.nbphe.org/about/

National Board of Public Health Examiners. (2023b). *CPH Content Outline*. https://www.nbphe.org/cph-content-outline/

National Board of Public Health Examiners. (2023c). *Eligibility Requirements*. https://www.nbphe.org/eligibility/

National Commission on Health Education Credentialing, Inc. (n.d.-a). *Continuing Education Requirements for CHES®*. https://www.nchec.org/ches-recertification

National Commission on Health Education Credentialing, Inc. (n.d.-b). *Continuing Education Requirements for MCHES®*. https://www.nchec.org/mches-recertification

National Commission for Health and Education Credentialing, Inc. (2020). *Areas of Responsibility, Competencies and Sub-competencies for Health Education Specialist Practice Analysis II 2020 (HESPA II 2020)*. https://assets.speakcdn.com/assets/2251/hespa_competencies_and_sub-competencies_052020.pdf

Society for Public Health Education. (2023). *History*. https://www.sophe.org/about/history/

The National Board of Respiratory Care. (2023). *Asthma Educator Specialist (AE-C)*. https://www.nbrc.org/examinations/certified-asthma-educator-ae-c/

U.S. Department of Health and Human Services & Division of Adolescent and School Health, National Center for HIV/AIDS, Viral Hepatitis, STD, and TB Prevention. (2022). *Professional Development*. https://www.cdc.gov/healthyyouth/professional_development/index.htm#:~:text=Professional%20development%20contributes%20to%20this,that%20positively%20impact%20young%20people

U.S. Department of Health and Human Services & Office of Disease Prevention and Health Promotion. (2021). *About the Physical Activity Guidelines*. https://health.gov/our-work/nutrition-physical-activity/physical-activity-guidelines/about-physical-activity-guidelines

U.S. Department of Health and Human Services & Office of Disease Prevention and Health Promotion. (2023). *Campaign Materials*. https://health.gov/our-work/nutrition-physical-activity/move-your-way-community-resources/campaign-materials

Vanderbilt University. (2023). *Bloom's Taxonomy*. https://cft.vanderbilt.edu/guides-sub-pages/blooms-taxonomy/#:~:text=Familiarly%20known%20as%20Bloom's%20Taxonomy,Analysis%2C%20Synthesis%2C%20and%20Evaluation

Implications for the Future

DOI: 10.4324/9781003504320-10

Learning Objectives

After reading this chapter, learners will be able to:

- Identify trends in U.S. health data compared to other countries
- Describe the health care and public health systems in the United States
- Describe current challenges for the health education and promotion workforce
- Identify opportunities to implementing health promotion efforts

---

Keywords

- 10 Essential Services
- Affordable Care Act (ACA)
- Health Insurance Marketplace
- Infant Mortality Rate
- Influencer
- Life Expectancy
- Maternal Mortality Rate
- Medicare

- Return on Investment (ROI)
- Structural Racism and Discrimination (SRD)
- Thinking in Systems (TiS)
- Underinsured
- Uninsured
- Medicaid

Self-Reflection Question

Take a moment and reflect on these questions:

1. What are the current workplace challenges for HES?
2. What are the current leading health issues in the United States?
3. How can HES make a sustainable impact on leading health issues?

DOI: 10.4324/9781003504320-10

Ensuring HES are prepared to enter and stay in the public health workforce with accurate knowledge and skills is crucial to ensuring the health of communities. A competent and well-trained public health workforce is essential for several reasons, including preventing and controlling infectious and chronic diseases; managing public health emergencies, such as natural disasters or pandemics; promoting healthy lifestyles and behaviors; monitoring environmental hazards; developing health-promoting policies at local, state, and federal levels; and, conducting surveillance and research to identify trends in health data. A competent public health workforce works toward eliminating health disparities and promoting health equity in everything they do.

Public health professionals and HES must also consider global health challenges and their impact on individuals and communities on a daily basis. This work might include managing epidemics, such as obesity; responding to pandemics, such as COVID-19; participating in vaccine campaigns in efforts to control and eradicate some diseases; and, providing humanitarian aid during times of natural disasters or international conflict. Most importantly, HES and other public health professionals must do this work while building and maintaining public trust and confidence. Expertise and transparency in actions and communication are crucial for garnering the public's support and collaboration in everyday situations as well as during public health emergencies. This chapter will review the status of public health in the United States compared to other countries and identify future challenges and opportunities for HES and other professionals who work in public health.

Health Status of the United States

Despite spending far more on healthcare per capita than any other country, the United States lags behind on several important health indicators (Gunji et al., 2023). Specifically,

> ...health spending per person in the U.S. was nearly two times higher than in the closest country, Germany, and four times higher than in South Korea. In the U.S., that includes spending for people in public programs like Medicaid, the Children's Health Insurance Program, Medicare, and military plans; spending by those with private employer-sponsored coverage or other private insurance; and out-of-pocket health spending.
>
> *(Gunji et al., 2023, para. 7)*

Two important health indicators when determining the health of a nation are **infant mortality rates** (IMR) and **maternal mortality rates** (MMR). Despite being a high-income country, the United States falls short in protecting its youngest community members and those who are pregnant. The IMR and MMR are both higher in the United States, when compared to other developed nations. Gunji et al. (2023) reported an IMR of 5.4 (per 1,000 live births) and an MMR of 23.8 (per 100,000 live births) respectively, with the next closest countries at an IMR of 4.5 (Canada) and an MMR of 13.6 (New Zealand). Factors contributing to these discrepancies include several social determinants of health (SDOH), such as racism, lack of access to healthcare, socioeconomic inequality, and inadequate perinatal and pregnancy care. Countries that have lower infant and maternal mortality rates prioritize access to health programs and services, maternal and child health support, health promotion and education, and related safety nets. While the United States has made efforts to address these issues, the gaps in infant and maternal mortality rates emphasize the need for continued improvements in healthcare accessibility and equity.

Similarly, **life expectancy** in the United States, which had been increasing over several years, continues to be lower than in many other developed countries. According to Worldometer, which uses data from the United Nations Population Division, the United States ranks 46th (out of 201 countries) with a life expectancy of 79.74 for both sexes

> ### SIDEBAR: DID YOU KNOW?
>
> The Centers for Disease Control and Prevention (CDC) sponsors the Maternal, Infant, and Child Health Workgroup, which is a group of professionals who are experts in infant and maternal mortality and related topics (U.S. Department of Health and Human Services [USDHHS], n.d.). This Workgroup developed the Healthy People 2030 (HP 2030) objectives related to infant and maternal mortality and are charged with monitoring the data as the decade progresses (USDHHS, n.d.).
>
> To review the HP 2030 objectives on infant mortality, please visit https://tinyurl.com/mpchf47d. To review the HP 2030 objectives on maternal mortality, please visit https://tinyurl.com/2bbv35y5.

(2023). Hong Kong has the highest life expectancy at 85.83 (Worldometer, 2023). Switzerland, Canada and the United Kingdom also had life expectancies higher than the United States at 84.38, 83.02 and 82.31, respectively. Chad has the lowest life expectancy at 53.68 (Worldometer, 2023).

Contributors to the lower life expectancy in the United States include high rates of chronic diseases, unequal access to healthcare, and socioeconomic disparities. Kochanek et al. reported that between 2014 and 2017, the slight decline (0.3 years) in life expectancy in the United States was mostly due to increases in mortality due to unintentional injuries, Alzheimer's disease, and suicide (2020, para. 4). In addition, between 2017 and 2018, the slight (0.1) increase in life expectancy was due mostly to decreases in mortality from cancer, unintentional injuries, and chronic lower respiratory diseases (Kochanek et al., 2020, para. 5). Woolf examined life expectancy in the United States between 1933 and 2021 and identified key trends (2023). Overall, Woolf found that life expectancy in the United States has basically plateaued since 2010 while continuing to increase in most other countries (2023). During the early years of the COVID-19 pandemic, the United States had the largest drop in life expectancy in the world except for two countries, Bulgaria and Slovakia (Woolf, 2023). Woolf offers many possible reasons for this overall decline over the decades, but suggests that an increase in conservative policies that affect health may be to blame – noting that states in the South Central and Midwest have the slowest growth in life expectancy (2023). In the United States, some of the same issues listed as factors driving high infant and maternal mortality, such as universal healthcare systems, improved access to preventive care, and social safety nets, are factors in a lower life expectancy. HES and others in public health are working on these issues, yet despite their efforts – disparities persist. This emphasizes the critical need for meaningful and sustained investment in public health programs and services.

Activity 10.1: Discussion

In early 2022, Health Affairs interviewed Harriet A. Washington, the author of the popular book *Medical Apartheid: The Dark History of Medical Experimentation on Black Americans from Colonial Times to the Present.* Please watch the 30-minute interview at https://www.youtube.com/watch?v=YVPFUlRAgUU and consider your responses to the following questions:

1. What stood out to you about the historical information that was shared about anti-Black racism in medicine and research?
2. What is your reaction to the information shared on the lack of informed consent historically and the concerns that were raised about practices that perpetuate a lack of informed consent today?
3. Does exploring the topic of racism and health impact your thoughts on the role of HES and public health professionals today? If yes, how?
4. Does the information shared in the video impact your view of how HES should build and maintain trust with Black and African American communities? If yes, how?

Social Determinants of Health

Have you ever heard that your zip code determines your health? It's true. The reality is that the zip code where you were born and live can have a significant impact on health outcomes. Research demonstrates that people from two different zip codes that are right next to each other can have very different health outcomes and, therefore, a different life expectancy (Orminski, 2021). Factors such as access to quality healthcare, nutritious food, safe housing, and educational opportunities can vary widely from one neighborhood to another. In disadvantaged, vulnerable, or marginalized communities, residents often face higher rates of chronic diseases, limited access to healthcare, and increased exposure to environmental hazards. These disparities in resources and opportunities can result in substantial disparities between individuals living in different zip codes. According to Orminski, where an individual lives is perhaps the most important contributor to their health and life expectancy (2021). Orminski states that "...up to 60% of your health is determined solely by your zip code" (2021, para. 1). The environment, both social and built, where someone lives, works, plays, and prays may have more of an impact on their health than lifestyle behaviors and even genetics.

SIDEBAR: DID YOU KNOW?

The CDC developed a tool called PLACES, in collaboration with the Robert Wood Johnson foundation and the CDC Foundation, for users to search for specific health data across the country. PLACES generates population-level data analysis and provides estimates of health measures for counties, census tracts, and zip codes throughout the United States. The tool is designed to assist "...local health departments and jurisdictions, regardless of population size and rurality, to better understand the burden and geographic distribution of health measures in their areas and assist them in planning public health interventions" (Centers for Disease Control and Prevention [CDC], 2023b, para. 1).

Activity 10.2: Practice your Skills

Review the PLACES website at https://www.cdc.gov/places/index.html and complete the following steps:

1. Select the *Comparison Report* button and build a report that includes five neighboring counties by selecting *Add County.* You will need to select a state and then choose from the list of counties from the pop-up menu. You can choose your own state and the neighboring counties to where you attend school or live, for example.
2. Review the data for each county in comparison to the U.S. data.
3. Compare the data between the five counties you selected.
4. Answer the following questions:

   a. What are some of the differences in health outcomes between the counties?
   b. Which county is the healthiest? How did you determine that?
   c. Were you surprised by what you learned in this activity about the 5 counties?
   d. How might you address the differences in health outcomes between the counties if you worked for the state health department?

Next, please visit https://www.cdc.gov/places/social-determinants-of-health-and-places-data/index.html and open one of the available data sets listed towards the end of the page and review the information.

After reviewing the dataset that contains SDOH data, answer the following questions:

1. What specific data are available in the dataset you selected?
2. How might a HES use the data in the dataset that you chose?
3. What is the SDOH data for the five counties you researched in the PLACES tool helpful to know?

For example, differences in life expectancy vary greatly between zip codes in Washington, DC. The life expectancy difference between 20088 (with the longest life expectancy at 96.1 years) and 20020 (with the shortest life expectancy at 63.2) is 32.9 years (Minor, 2020; Owens-Young, 2023). This difference is significant and it is difficult to learn because the actual distance between these two zip codes is less than ten miles. This disparity in life expectancy highlights how different health outcomes can be affected just by the environment where people live because of "...the air we breathe, the food we eat, the services we have access to, the opportunities afforded to us" (Minor, 2020, para. 3). These SDOH of air quality, access to foods, and access to healthcare services and well-paying jobs all reveal that disparities in our communities reflect decades of **Structural Racism and Discrimination** (SRD). SRD refers to

...conditions (e.g. residential segregation and institutional policies) that limit opportunities, resources, power, and well-being of individuals and populations based on race/ethnicity and other statuses, including but not limited to:

Gender
Sexual orientation

Gender identity
Disability status
Social class or socioeconomic status
Religion
National origin
Immigration status
Limited English proficiency
Physical characteristics or health conditions

(National Institutes of Health, 2023, para. 1–3)

Neighborhood characteristics, such as food deserts, low income, underfunded school systems, polluted air, and unsafe drinking water, are all found more frequently in areas where more Black households are located (Minor, 2020). Addressing these issues is a fundamental job function for HES and every professional in public health. It requires intentional, comprehensive efforts, including programs, services, and policies that promote health equity along with the understanding that a person's health is deeply intertwined with the environment in which they live. Breaking this link between zip code and health and dismantling structural racism in the United States are crucial steps toward achieving health equity for all.

Activity 10.3: Discussion

Unnatural Causes: Is inequality making us sick? is a four-hour PBS documentary series that explores the root causes of socio-economic and racial health disparities. In episode three of the series, the concept of the *Latino Paradox* is explored (California Newsreel, 2008). The Latino Paradox, also called Hispanic Paradox, describes the phenomenon that

> [r]ecent Mexican immigrants, although poorer, tend to be healthier than the average American. They have lower rates of death, heart disease, cancer, and other illnesses, despite being less educated, earning less and having the stress of adapting to a new country and a new language.
>
> *(California Newsreel, 2008, para. 1)*

Protective factors such as cultural traditions and strong social networks may play a significant role in helping through the stress of immigration (California Newsreel, 2008). Sadly, "[a]fter five years or more in the U.S., they are 1.5 times more likely to have high blood pressure – and be obese – than when they arrived. Within one generation, their health is as poor as other Americans of similar income status" (California Newsreel, 2008, para. 2).

To learn more about the documentary, please visit https://unnaturalcauses.org/.

Health Care and Public Health Systems in the United States

The healthcare system in the United States is a complex and multi-faceted structure with many layers. Unlike most developed countries, the U.S. healthcare system is primarily a combination of public and private sectors. It relies on a system of individual health insurance, where people often secure coverage through employers or government programs, like **Medicare** and **Medicaid**. While this system has the potential to offer high quality medical care, it faces significant challenges. One of the most concerning issues is the high cost of healthcare, which places an unnecessary financial burden on many Americans. Access to healthcare varies, with disparities in access to care and thus health outcomes too often related to socioeconomic status and geographical location. Health advocates, including elected officials, have worked diligently toward achieving healthcare reform to address all of these issues and make healthcare more accessible and affordable, and some progress in this area has happened with the passing of the Affordable Care Act. However, the debate over the best approach to healthcare continues, and the struggle to find the best options for ensuring quality, accessible, and affordable healthcare in the United States ensues.

Federal Public Health System

The public health system in the United States is a network of government agencies and organizations at the federal, state, and local levels that are designed to work together to protect and improve the health of the population. Agencies within the federal government (as indicated in Table 10.1) include the U.S. Department of Health and Human Services (HHS), which oversees the Centers for Disease Control and Prevention (CDC), the Food and Drug Administration (FDA), the Centers for Medicare and Medicaid (CMS), the Agency for Healthcare Research and Quality (AHRQ), the Substance Abuse and Mental Health Administration (SAMHSA), the National Institutes of Health (NIH), and others. Another federal agency related to health is the Environmental Protection Agency (EPA). These agencies are key components to the public health system at the federal level.

This network of agencies and organizations encompass a wide range of functions and activities aimed at preventing and responding to short-term and long-term health threats, promoting health and wellness, and ensuring that communities have access to essential health services. Public health emphasizes preventive measures such as vaccinations, screenings, and health education to reduce the incidence of diseases at all levels, and public health programs and services can occur in a wide range of settings, including communities, schools, workplaces, and government agencies.

Table 10.1 Examples of Federal Public Health Agencies

Agency Name	Agency Website
U.S. Department of Health and Human Services (HHS)	https://www.hhs.gov/
Centers for Disease Control and Prevention (CDC)	https://www.cdc.gov/
Food and Drug Administration (FDA)	https://www.fda.gov/
Centers for Medicare and Medicaid (CMS)	https://www.cms.gov/
Agency for Healthcare Research and Quality (AHRQ)	https://www.ahrq.gov/
Substance Abuse and Mental Health Administration (SAMHSA)	https://www.samhsa.gov/
National Institutes of Health (NIH)	https://www.nih.gov/
Environmental Protection Agency (EPA)	https://www.epa.gov/

Activity 10.4: Discussion

To learn more about how HHS is organized and which additional federal agencies support public health, please visit https://www.hhs.gov/about/agencies/orgchart/index.html to view the organizational chart. Each agency name is hyperlinked. Review each agency for what they are responsible for, including their organizational chart. Then share your responses to the following questions:

1. What role does each agency play in protecting the public's health?
2. What do you think are some of the skills needed to work in these agencies?
3. Could HES support the mission of each of these agencies? How?
4. Are there agencies that you might be interested in as a potential future employer?

State and Local Public Health System

At the state level, there is a state health department responsible for implementing health programs and policies, monitoring health trends, and responding to public health emergencies within the state. The same applies to the five U.S. territories and three freely associated states. The five U.S. territories include American Samoa, Commonwealth of the Northern Mariana Islands, Guam, Puerto Rico, and U.S. Virgin Islands (Association of State and Territorial Health Officials [ASTHO], 2023). The three freely associated states include Federated States of Micronesia, The Republic of the Marshall Islands, and The Republic of Palau (ASTHO, 2023).

At the local level, local health departments serve cities and counties within each state. They provide important public health services, such as vaccinations, disease surveillance, environmental health inspections, and health education. Additional programs might include monitoring for new and emerging infectious diseases, prevention and management of chronic conditions, ensuring maternal and child health, and emergency planning and preparedness. At the local public health level, boards of health are administrative bodies that are elected or appointed to lead, guide, and support the coordination

SIDEBAR: DID YOU KNOW?

To assist local and state public health, there are two organizations that provide support, technical assistance, networking opportunities, advocacy support, access to research, and high quality resources at the national level. These are the National Association of City and County Health Officials (NACCHO) for local health departments and the Association of State and Territorial Health Officials (ASTHO) for the 50 state health departments and the health departments for the five territories and three freely associated states.

To learn more about each of these organizations, please visit https://www.naccho.org/ and https://www.astho.org/.

SIDEBAR: DID YOU KNOW?

There are similarities and differences between state and local health departments. To learn more, please review this document prepared by the Public Health Law Center https://publichealthlawcenter.org/sites/default/files/resources/phlc-fs-state-local-reg-authority-publichealth-2015_0.pdf and implementation of public health programs and services. Some responsibilities of boards of health can include reviewing and proposing public health regulations, policies, and priorities; overseeing the implementation of CHAs and CHIPs; participating in strategic planning; and collaborating with other health entities in the community.

10 Essential Services. In 1994, the **10 Essential Public Health Services** (EPHS) was developed as a guide for communities to support public health services in collaboration with local and state health departments (CDC, 2023a). The list was revised in 2020 through a combined effort of public health leaders, the Public Health National Center for Innovations (PHNCI), and the de Beaumont Foundation to "bring the framework in line with current and future public health practice" (CDC, 2023a, para. 1). Specifically, this list provides a framework to protect and promote the health of all people in all communities by ensuring that "conditions that enable optimal health for all and seek to remove systemic and structural barriers that have resulted in health inequities" (CDC 2023a, para. 3). The services are organized into three main categories: assessment, policy development and assurance. Across these three categories are services such as assessing and monitoring population health, communicating to inform and educate community members, and building a diverse and skilled workforce (as indicated in Figure 10.1).

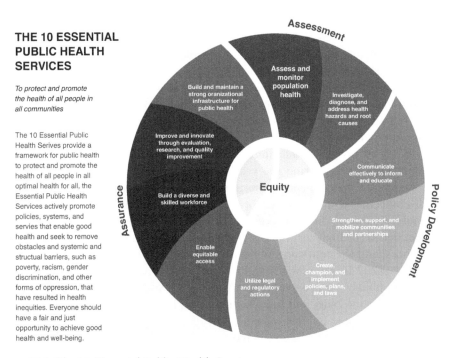

Figure 10.1 The 10 Essential Public Health Services

Note: This image was produced by Public Health National Center for Innovations on September 9, 2020 and is included in the 10 Essential Public Health Services Toolkit available for use in the public domain available at https://www.cdc.gov/publichealthgateway/publichealthservices/essentialhealthservices.html

Activity 10.5: Practice Your Skills

1. Make a chart that lists each of the ten Essential Public Health Services indicated in Figure 10.1 (in this chapter).
2. Next to each of the ten Essential Public Health Services listed, add the job responsibilities from the job description that most closely matches it.

Once the chart is complete, respond to the following questions:

1. Do any of the ten Essential Services have more than one job responsibility listed?
2. Are there any of the ten Essential Services that do not have any job responsibilities listed?
3. What would a job description for a HES need to include to have each of the ten Essential Services addressed?

Healthcare Systems

While public health institutions and professionals play an important role in promoting health and preventing diseases at the population level, hospitals and primary healthcare providers (sometimes called PCPs) are integral to the delivery of healthcare to individuals. This clinical care is delivered within hospitals, urgent care centers, and at individual offices of healthcare providers.

In 2022, 92.1% of all people in the United States had health insurance at one point during the year (Keisler-Starkey et al., 2023). Healthcare insurance is coverage frequently offered by employers, but many people may need to purchase insurance individually. Keisler-Starkey et al. reported that in that same year, 54.4% had health insurance through their employer while 9.9% purchased it directly on the **health insurance marketplace** (2023). Healthcare insurance plans vary widely in terms of coverage, costs, and available provider networks. However, there are also many people who are **uninsured** or **underinsured** and therefore cannot access healthcare when needed. In 2022, 10.8% of people in the United States between the ages of 19 and 64 were uninsured at some point during the year (Keisler-Starkey et al., 2023). Despite the fact that the United States spends more than any other country per capita on healthcare, health outcomes continue to be worse than other developed countries (Ducharme, 2023). In addition, more than 70% of Americans believe that the healthcare system is failing them due to the high cost of healthcare and insurance, the difficulty in accessing needed services, and the confusing administrative barriers of the health insurance system (Ducharme, 2023). Along with employer and marketplace-based health insurance, there are two publicly funded programs: Medicare, which provides health insurance for people aged 65 and older and some younger people with disabilities, and Medicaid, which provides coverage for low-income individuals and families. However, both of these programs can be challenging to navigate given the types of benefits available, determining eligibility, navigating rules and restrictions and restrictions, and finding providers who accept them (Ali, 2020; Walker & Gorenstein, 2023).

The **Affordable Care Act** (ACA), signed into law in 2010, introduced insurance marketplaces where individuals can compare and purchase health insurance plans without needing employer-sponsored coverage (Healthcare.gov, n.d.). It also included the individual mandate, which requires most Americans to obtain health insurance

(Healthcare.gov, n.d.). ACA was designed to increase the number of people in the United States who are covered by health insurance and to make health insurance more affordable. The ACA provides subsidies that lower the costs of health insurance for people living between 100% and 400% of the federal poverty level (Healthcare.gov, n.d.). The ACA was also designed to expand Medicaid to more people, although not all states participate in this expansion, as well as encourage programs and services that work to lower the cost of healthcare overall (Healthcare.gov, n.d.).

Hospitals and hospital systems are large medical facilities and organizations that provide a wide range of inpatient and outpatient services, including emergency care, surgery, diagnostic procedures, and specialized screenings and treatments. They are focused on providing direct medical care and treatment to individuals, often in an acute or emergency setting. Physicians, nurse practitioners, and other healthcare professionals offer primary care services, including preventive care and basic medical treatment. Other healthcare professionals, called specialists, have expertise in specific medical fields, such as cardiology, oncology, or neurology. While hospitals and healthcare providers are integral to the delivery of individual healthcare services, public health institutions and professionals play a broader role in promoting health and preventing diseases at the population level. Both components are essential for a comprehensive and effective healthcare system.

Thinking in Systems (TiS). A career in health education and promotion and public health is guaranteed to be an exciting journey. The skills that HES bring to communities and employers are incredibly diverse, transferable to multiple settings, and can be applied to complex challenges. This is in large part because public health professionals think and work through complex issues with a Thinking in Systems (TiS) approach (CDC, 2021b). Thinking in Systems (TiS) is a framework that

> ...help[s] public health professionals think more effectively, and systemically, about the issues they face. This can lead to identifying possible policy solutions that may not have been readily apparent, which can be helpful in the realm of using policy to improve the health and wellbeing of populations.
>
> *(CDC, 2021b, para. 1)*

Approaching public health challenges by thinking about the systems involved is challenging and requires a specific and logical approach. The CDC describes systems as "the elements that work together to generate the results you want or desire to change. The system is the interplay between: policies and procedures, infrastructure, spending decisions, human actions, and intangible drivers of behavior (e.g., trust, goodwill, etc.)" (2021a, para. 2). Knowing how these systems impact each other is necessary for systems change to occur. Typically, change is necessary when a system problem occurs. System problems generally share four distinct characteristics (CDC, 2021a). Systems problems evolve and are constantly changing, they impact diverse groups of people with specific needs and interests, "dependencies between individuals, organizations, regions, etc. exist and are important," and "they can be hard to describe" (CDC, 2021a, para. 4). According to Yphantides et al. (2015), "[t]he 'systems perspective,' broadly defined, has enabled public health to break out of the siloed role in which it had been typically viewed in the US to become interdisciplinary, inter-agency, and inter-organizational" (para. 13). Therefore, HES and other public health professionals have to consider the implications of their work, utilize their skills in assessing needs, and apply their knowledge of behavioral health theories, program planning models, and evaluation.

Role of Education in Public Health

HES can be employed in multiple settings. Regardless of the setting, they have the responsibility to educate individuals about health. By teaching new skills and knowledge, HES are tasked with improving health outcomes. This may be helping someone quit using tobacco, teaching someone how to prepare meals with less fat and sugar or training someone on how to monitor their blood sugar. Hahn and Truman emphasize the important role of education in improving health (2015). They state that "...education – the product and personal attribute acquired – is both a critical component of a person's health and a contributing cause of other elements of the person's concurrent and future health" (para. 7). Knowledge is power and with knowledge about health comes the ability to make informed choices about our health. Being educated about our health has the potential to positively affect health equity. Hahn and Truman argue that being educated is a component of being healthy and that with increased education comes improved health (2015). Thus, providing health education and promotion programs and services creates one upstream solution to a root cause of poor health.

Activity 10.6: Practice your Skills

Whether a HES is early, mid, or advanced level in their career, it can be incredibly helpful to meet other HES and public health professionals. These colleagues can provide support, share resources, and help HES get connected to others in the field. Some suggestions to find HES and other public health professionals include:

1. Join public health LinkedIn groups, such as the *American Public Health* and *Public Health Professionals* group.
2. Engage with a local chapter of the Society for Public Health Education. To learn more, please visit https://www.sophe.org/membership/sophe-chapters/.
3. Sign up for a listserv with a focus on public health. For example, if you want to connect with other HES and public health professionals committed to ending health inequities, then you may want to sign up to join the *The Spirit of 1848* listserv. To learn more, please visit http://www.spiritof1848.org/. If you are planning to or work in the environmental health sector, then you may want to sign up for the Environmental Health Services listserv. To learn more, please visit https://www.cdc.gov/nceh/ehs/listserv/listserv.htm.

Current Challenges to Implementing Health Education and Promotion

The implementation of health education and promotion programs can face several challenges that impact the ability of the program to be effective and reach the intended audiences. These challenges include limited resources, political influences, social media, and the public health workforce.

Limited Resources

Funding constraints can restrict the development and implementation of effective health education and promotion programs. Adequate financial support, from agencies such as the CDC, is crucial for conducting research, creating impactful campaigns, and sustaining long-term educational initiatives. The Trust for America's Health (The Trust) reports that

> ...while the United States spends an estimated $3.6 trillion annually on health, less than 3 percent of that spending is directed toward public health and prevention. Furthermore, public health spending as a proportion of total health spending has been decreasing since 2000 and falling in inflation-adjusted terms since the Great Recession. Health departments across the country are battling 21st-century health threats with 20th century resources. The COVID-19 crisis demonstrates this reality in the starkest of terms.
>
> *(para. 3, 2023)*

The trust also reports that CDC's budget is close to where it was in 2008 after adjusting for inflation indicating that the budget has not kept up with current needs such as fighting obesity, and preparing for emergencies (2023). In addition, the Prevention and Public Health Fund, which was planned to increase the nation's funding in public health initiatives, remains at half of what it should have been in 2020 due to monies being diverted to other programs (Trust for America's Health, 2023). A specific example of this is how much the United States spends to control and prevent tobacco use as compared to the marketing of tobacco by tobacco companies. The United States spends $241 billion on healthcare costs related to tobacco use annually (Campaign for Tobacco-Free Kids [CTFK], 2023). While the tobacco industry spends $8.6 billion in marketing their products in the United States (CTFK, 2023), states spend a meager $330.0 million in tobacco prevention and control efforts (CDC 2022a, 2022b).

Political Influences

In the United States, political influence can and often does play a significant role in deciding public health policies, priorities, and outcomes. The decisions made by elected officials, policymakers, and government institutions have far-reaching effects on the health of a population. This can happen through environmental policy decisions, rules, and regulations on eligibility of healthcare programs and services, funding decisions, global collaborations, as well management or mismanagement of public health crises. Bias argues that "...public health is *always* political" (2020). While most federal funding for public health in the United States receives bipartisan support, many specific public health programs do not. For example, soda taxes, needle exchange programs, universal health insurance, and vaccination initiatives do not (Bias, 2020). Some recent examples of health challenges that faced extra scrutiny from the political system include the COVID-19 response, reproductive health, and the effects of climate change on health. Although advocates for public health rely on science and evidence-based research to inform the development and implementation of health programs and services, the evidence can often be the center of heated debates. Because HES and other public health professionals often work with elected officials to provide subject matter expertise, understanding and resisting political pressures are important skills to have to carry forward needed health programs and services.

Social Media

The rise of social media, while having many benefits, also poses some challenges for HES. **Influencers** on social media often share their personal opinions rather than facts about prominent health issues. Because social media influencers are often paid by sponsors, their content may or may not be their own nor accurate. Suarez-Lledo and Alvarez-Galvez reported that misinformation about health topics, including smoking products, marijuana and the human papillomavirus vaccine, is quite common on social media (2021). Other topics that have been addressed with incorrect information have included dieting, spread of infectious diseases, and cancer (Suarez-Lledo & Alvarez-Galvez, 2021). Competing messages from various sources, including respected health organizations and agencies to social media platforms, can dilute the impact and effectiveness of health education campaigns. Ramakrishnan reported that "...more than 70% of Americans have been exposed to medical misinformation, of which 82% has come from social media" (2022, para. 2). Additionally, Ramakrishnan shared that, "... 44% of respondents weren't confident in deciphering whether the medical information they consumed was accurate or not" (para. 3). This requires that HES remain informed about the kinds of inaccurate information that is being shared and develop appropriate responses through social media posts with correct information through their organization's platforms or as programs that offer correct information and support to make healthy behavior changes possible.

Activity 10.7: Discussion

The Academy of Nutrition and Dietetics, a professional association of over 100,000 dietitians and nutritionists, is considered one of the most influential professional health associations in the United States. Because of this, their endorsement of products can lead to increased sales and profits for food companies. Recent research on this association shows that it receives substantial funding from companies such as the National Dairy Council, Coca-Cola, PepsiCo, General Mills, Kelloggs, and Kraft (Malkan, 2023). To learn more about this practice and its implications, please read the following two articles and share your responses to the questions.

https://tinyurl.com/m96623xh

https://tinyurl.com/2v6v35xm

1. What is the mission of the Academy of Nutrition and Dietetics?
2. Who are the primary funders of the Academy of Nutrition and Dietetics?
3. Does their mission align with the goals of some of the companies that fund the Academy?
4. Do you believe that there are any conflicts of interest with the funding source for the Academy of Nutrition and Dietetics? Why or why not?

Public Health Workforce

A final challenge to examine is that of the public health workforce itself. With the impact of COVID-19 on the workforce and with many people nearing retirement age, there has been a reduction in the number of people working in public health (Leider et al., 2023). In fact, Leider et al. report that in 2017, 61% of state public health employees planned to leave or retire within the next five years and by 2021, and 49% had left (2023). Big cities and local public health saw similar declines in that same time period, with 55%, 51% and 53%, 51%, respectively (Leider et al., 2023). In addition, many healthcare workers are reporting burnout, especially as a result of the COVID-19 pandemic (USDHHS, 2022). Reasons for burnout include mental health challenges, workloads and scheduling issues, administrative hurdles, and overall lack of support (USDHHS, 2022). The COVID-19 pandemic was stressful to many in healthcare, particularly due to the political and economic pressures that occurred. Current efforts to address this burnout include increasing access to mental health programs and services, increasing social support, addressing racism and bias in the workplace, and committing to a culture of health and safety for all healthcare workers (USDHHS, 2022). In addition, in a recent Public Health Workforce Interests and Needs Survey that focused on COVID-19 related work, 56% of the public health workforce reported post-traumatic stress disorder, 41% of public health executives felt bullied or threatened, and one in three have considered leaving the field (deBeaumont Foundation, 2022). Despite this, there was some good news that came out of the survey: 79% reported overall satisfaction with their jobs (deBeaumont Foundation, 2022). Although implementing effective health education and promotion programs has some serious challenges, current and future HES need to both be aware of and willing to work on overcoming these challenges in an effort to improve population health.

> **SIDEBAR: DID YOU KNOW?**
>
> Every community has health challenges; however, communities have different resources and capacity to address them. Those who work in rural settings will benefit from the Rural Health Promotion and Disease Prevention Toolkit from the Rural Health Information Hub.
>
> To review toolkit, please visit https://www.ruralhealthinfo.org/toolkits/health-promotion.

Activity 10.8: Discussion

Are you looking for a high-quality documentary that is interesting to watch and takes a deep-dive into the system issues and challenges with public health and medicine? Then you may be interested in the compiled list from the University of Otago, Wellington designed for medical students that includes 35 top-rated documentaries (2023).

To learn which documentaries made the list and what to consider for your next movie night, please visit https://tinyurl.com/4pnjekjk.

Concepts in Action 10.1

Background: *Tasha* (she/her) likes to reflect on how she has made an impact in her community.

Tasha's father died at the age of 47, when she was only 12 years old. His death was a shock to the whole family and Tasha wanted a career that could prevent something like this happening to someone else. Tasha's father died of a heart attack. He actually had a family history of heart health issues, but that was only discovered after he died. He did not go to the doctor often, despite pleas from Tasha's mother. Tasha learned in school that men are less likely to visit the doctor and that got her really excited to have a career to change that. As a HES, Tasha works hard to understand challenges and barriers to accessing quality health care. She works hard to stay on top of the latest science about men's health and heart health. Tasha's decision to become a HES has been an exciting and challenging one. Being a HES requires patience, steadfast diligence, and a commitment to the work. When Tasha was interviewed for the alumni association at the university that she attended, she shared

> … I am so proud of the work I do every day in the role that I have. It requires that I build trust with others and promote evidence-based strategies to make improvements in health outcomes. I believe it is such an important field of work and I am excited for all the possibilities that it offers. I know my dad would be proud that I am helping to change the way we think about health and that I get to educate people about health and the impact of the environment in which we live. Recently I was part of a Task Force in the city where I was raised to promote walking and biking with paved sidewalks and walkways through the downtown and midtown areas. To see so many people walking and biking makes me so happy. I really do recommend anyone who wants to make a difference in health to consider a career as a HES.

Opportunities to Implementing Public Health Promotion Efforts

Despite the challenges, opportunities for public health interventions in the United States are endless. There are opportunities to continue to build on the foundation of successful health promotion programs and policies, work toward health equity, leverage technology, and promote the return on investments in public health. HES and others working in public health are engaged and ready to improve population health while addressing ongoing challenges.

Foundation of Success

Public health has celebrated many achievements over the past 120 years, including, but is not limited to, decreased cases, deaths, and healthcare costs from vaccine-preventable diseases; improved control of infectious diseases, cancer, and cardiovascular diseases; continued tobacco control efforts and advances in emergency preparedness and planning (CDC, 2011). By focusing on preventive measures such as vaccinations, screenings, and health education, public health interventions can and do reduce the incidence of both infectious and chronic diseases while enhancing overall health and well-being. Promoting prevention not only improves individual and population health outcomes but also contributes to more effective and efficient use of the healthcare system by reducing the need for treatments and interventions. This strong foundation of success is a reminder of how effective public health can be.

Working Towards Health Equity

Another key opportunity for HES is the promotion of health equity. Although disparities in health outcomes persist among different demographic groups in the United States, public health interventions that address the root causes of disparities, such as education, income and racism, can help create a more equitable healthcare system. Targeted interventions can focus on increasing access to healthcare services, improving educational opportunities, and addressing systemic factors that contribute to health inequities. Among other initiatives, HES can make an impact on health equity by helping to stop the spread of COVID-19, implementing programs and services that will address the opioid and substance use epidemics, strengthening community safety, and ensuring that policies are inclusive and designed to end racial inequities (Rosenthal et al., 2022).

Leveraging Technology

Social media and digital health technologies provide additional opportunities for HES to reach more people with health education and health promotion programs and campaigns. Mobile apps, wearable devices, and telehealth platforms are being utilized now more than ever and they offer innovative and accessible ways to reach individuals looking to improve their health. Public health campaigns leveraging these technologies can promote healthy behaviors, track health metrics, and facilitate communication between individuals and healthcare providers, fostering a more connected and collaborative approach to healthcare. Public health interventions also have the opportunity to address mental health challenges, which have gained increased recognition in recent years, and especially since COVID-19. Programs and services focusing on mental health education, reducing stigma, and expanding access to mental health services can make significant improvements in the mental health and well-being of the population. Because the United States continues to face ongoing and complex public health issues such as substance abuse, obesity, and chronic and infectious diseases, comprehensive approaches that combine education, environmental and policy changes, and community engagement can help mitigate these challenges and promote healthier lifestyles.

Promoting Return on Investments
Finally, there are opportunities to sell the concepts of public health. Effective health education and promotion programs need resources, both financial and human. By using return on investment (ROI) data, HES and others in public health can make the case for their work. For example, the Real Cost campaign, which was designed to prevent youth from using tobacco, has shown an ROI of $128 saved for every $1 spent (MacMonegle et al., 2018). The campaign cost about $250 million but is estimated to have saved $731 billion in health care costs. MacMonegle et al. also estimate that the campaign prevented over 175,000 youth from becoming regular tobacco users (2018). Similarly, Nianogo et al. found that for every dollar spent in the Women, Infants and Children (WIC) federal supplemental food and nutrition program, $2.48 was saved in future healthcare costs (2019). By using data such as these, HES can help to justify the resources needed to implement programs.

A Call to Action
There is a need for passionate people with specific skills in needs assessment, evaluation, program planning, advocacy, communication, leadership, and with a commitment to continuous professional development. Making an impact in the community as a HES is not only possible but also critical.

Summary
- Trends in U.S. health data show significantly worse health outcomes as compared to other similar countries, despite spending more per capita on healthcare. The infant mortality rate, maternal mortality rate and life expectancy are examples of health measures that require attention and action. SDOH contribute to these outcomes, including zip code and neighborhood.
- The healthcare and public health systems in the United States are complex and can be confusing. Lack of universal healthcare makes obtaining and effectively utilizing health insurance difficult for many. Federal, state, and local health agencies provide the foundation of public health services in the United States and are guided by the 10 Essential Health Services.
- Current challenges for HES include the cost of implementing comprehensive campaigns, current political climate, influence of social media, and the changing public health workforce. Since before the COVID-19 pandemic, many in the field are approaching retirement and reported feeling stressed and burned out. Support for healthcare workers is needed to ensure a capable workforce is available and prepared for the next public health crisis.
- As public health continues to emerge from COVID-19, there are opportunities that can assist HES implementing health promotion efforts. HES can build upon the many successes of the past 20 years, including improvements in tobacco control, emergency planning and preparedness and prevention of cancer and cardiovascular disease. Tools such as social media and return on investment data can also help to move public health forward.

■ **Health Insurance Explained – The YouToons Have It Covered**

  https://www.youtube.com/watch?v=-58VD3z7ZiQ

  This 5-minute and 24-second video from the Kaiser Family Foundation offers an overview of health insurance in the United States.

■ **Joy in Work Toolkit**

  https://www.naccho.org/uploads/downloadable-resources/JOY-IN-WORK-TOOLKIT-VFINAL-7-20-22.pdf

  This toolkit, developed by the National Association of City and County Health Officials, provides practical tips and strategies for engaging employees and improving work conditions and satisfaction.

■ **Support for Public Health Workers and Health Professionals from CDC**

  https://www.cdc.gov/mentalhealth/public-health-workers/index.html

  The CDC website contains multiple links for public health and health professionals on mental health, stress, resilience, and where to go for help.

References

Ali, R. (2020). *Making Medicare More Navigable*. https://www.commonwealthfund.org/blog/2020/making-medicare-more-navigable

American Public Health Association. (2013). *The Definition and Practice of Public Health Nursing: A Statement of the Public Health Nursing Section*. Washington, DC. https://www.apha.org/~/media/files/pdf/membergroups/phn/nursingdefinition.ashx

Association of State and Territorial Health Officials. (2023). *Territories and Freely Associated States*. https://www.astho.org/topic/territories-freely-associated-states/

Bias, T. (2020). *Public Health is Always Political*. Think Global Health. https://www.thinkglobalhealth.org/article/public-health-always-political

California Newsreel. (2008). *Episode Descriptions*. https://unnaturalcauses.org/episode_descriptions.php?page=3

Campaign for Tobacco-Free Kids. (2023). *The Toll of Tobacco in the United States*. https://www.tobaccofreekids.org/problem/toll-us

Centers for Disease Control and Prevention. (2011, May, 20). Ten great public health achievements – United States, 2001–2010. *Morbidity and Mortality Weekly, 60*(19), 619–623. https://www.cdc.gov/mmwr/preview/mmwrhtml/mm6019a5.htm

Centers for Disease Control and Prevention. (2021a). *How Do You Identify a Systems Problem?* https://www.cdc.gov/policy/polaris/tis/systems-problems/index.html

Centers for Disease Control and Prevention. (2021b). *Thinking in Systems Overview*. https://www.cdc.gov/policy/polaris/tis/index.html

Centers for Disease Control and Prevention. (2022a). *Costs and Expenditures*. https://www.cdc.gov/tobacco/data_statistics/fact_sheets/fast_facts/cost-and-expenditures.html

Centers for Disease Control and Prevention. (2022b). *National Tobacco Control Program Funding*. https://www.cdc.gov/tobacco/stateandcommunity/tobacco-control/program-funding/index.htm

Centers for Disease Control and Prevention. (2023a). *10 Essential Public Health Services*. https://www.cdc.gov/publichealthgateway/publichealthservices/essentialhealthservices.html

Centers for Disease Control and Prevention. (2023b). *Places: Local Data for Better Health*. https://www.cdc.gov/places/index.html

deBeaumont Foundation. (2022). *Rising Stress and Burnout in Public Health: Results of a National Survey of the Public Health Workforce*. https://debeaumont.org/wp-content/uploads/dlm_uploads/2022/03/Stress-and-Burnout-Brief_final.pdf

Ducharme, J. (2023). *Exclusive: More Than 70% of Americans Feel Failed by the Health Care System*. Time Magazine. https://time.com/6279937/us-health-care-system-attitudes/

Gunji, M.Z., Gumas, E.D., & Williams II, R.D. (2023). *U.S. Health Care from a Global Perspective, 2022: Accelerating Spending, Worsening Outcomes*. https://doi.org/10.26099/8ejy-yc74

Hahn, R.A. & Truman, B.I. (2015). Education improves public health and promotes health equity. *International Journal of Health Services, 45*(4), 657–678. https://doi.org/10.1177/0020731415585986

Healthcare.gov. (n.d.). *Affordable Care Act (ACA)*. https://www.healthcare.gov/glossary/affordable-care-act/

Keisler-Starkey, K., Bunch, L.N. & Lindstrom, R.A. (2023). United States Census Bureau. *Health Insurance Coverage in the United States: 2022*. https://www.census.gov/library/publications/2023/demo/p60-281.html#:~:text=Highlights,91.7%20percent%20or%20300.9%20million)

Kochanek, K.D., Anderson, R.N., & Arias, E. (2020). *Changes in Life Expectancy at Birth, 2010–2018*. NCHS Health E-Stat. https://www.cdc.gov/nchs/data/hestat/life-expectancy/life-expectancy-2018.htm

Leider, J.P., Castrucci, B.C., Robins, M., Bork, R.H., Fraser, M.R., Savoia, E., Piltch-Loeb, R., & Koh, H.K. (2023). The exodus of state and local public health employees: Separations started before and continued throughout COVID-19. *Health Affairs, 42*(3), 338–348. https://www.healthaffairs.org/doi/10.1377/hlthaff.2022.01251

MacMonegle, A.J., Nonnemaker, J., Duke, J.C., Farrelly, M.C., Zhao, X., Delahanty, J.C., Smith, A.A., Rao, P., & Allen, J.A. (2018). Cost-effectiveness analysis of the real cost campaign's effect on smoking prevention. *American Journal of Preventive Medicine, 55*(3), 319–325. https://www.ajpmonline.org/article/S0749-3797(18)31877-4/pdf

Malkan, S. (2023). *Academy of Nutrition and Dietetics: Corporate Capture of the Nutrition Profession*. https://usrtk.org/ultra-processed-foods/academy-of-nutrition-and-dietetics-corporate-capture-of-the-nutrition-profession/

Minor, L.B. (2020). *These 5 Numbers Tell You Everything You Need to Know about Racial Disparities in Health Care*. Fortune Magazine. https://fortune.com/2020/07/08/health-care-racism-zip-code-life-expectancy/

National Institutes of Health. (2023) *Structural Racism and Discrimination*. https://www.nimhd.nih.gov/resources/understanding-health-disparities/srd.html

Nianogo, R.A., Wang, M.C., Basurto-Davila, R., Nobari, T.Z., Prelip, M., Arah, O.A., & Whaley, S.E. (2019). Economic evaluation of California prenatal participation in the special supplemental nutrition program for women, infants and children (WIC) to prevent preterm birth. *Preventive Medicine, 124*, 42–49. https://www.sciencedirect.com/science/article/abs/pii/S0091743519301355?via%3Dihu, https://doi.org/10.1016/j.ypmed.2019.04.011

Orminski, E. (2021). National Community Reinvestment Coalition. *Your Zip Code Is More Important Than Your Genetic Code*. https://ncrc.org/your-zip-code-is-more-important-than-your-genetic-code/

Owens-Young, J. (2023). Blue Zones. *ZIP Code Effect: Neighborhood can Affect Life Expectancy by 30 Years*. https://www.bluezones.com/2020/02/zip-code-effect-your-neighborhood-determines-your-lifespan/

Ramakrishnan, A. (2022). The Atlanta Journal-Constitution. *Stop Taking Health Advice from Social Media Influencers*. https://www.ajc.com/pulse/stop-taking-health-advice-from-social-media-influencers/4E3S47KWFVHPBC5I6HHVP2RXEI/

Rosenthal, J., Rapfogel, N., & Johns, M. (2022). The Center for American Progress. *Top 10 Ways to Improve Health and Health Equity*. https://www.americanprogress.org/article/top-10-ways-to-improve-health-and-health-equity/

Suarez-Lledo, V. & Alvarez-Galvez, J. (2021). Prevalence of health misinformation on social media: Systematic review. *Journal of Medical Internet Research, 23*(1), e171–e87. https://doi.org/10.2196/17187

Trust for America's Health. (2023). *The Impact of Chronic Underfunding on America's Public Health System: Trends, Risks, and Recommendations, 2020*. https://www.tfah.org/report-details/publichealthfunding2020/

U.S. Department of Health and Human Services. (n.d.). *Maternal, Child, Infant and Maternal Health Workgroup*. Office of Disease Prevention and Health Promotion. https://health.gov/healthypeople/about/workgroups/maternal-infant-and-child-health-workgroup

U.S. Department of Health and Human Services, (2022). *The U.S. Surgeon General's Advisory on Building a Thriving Health Workforce*. United States Surgeon General. https://www.hhs.gov/surgeongeneral/priorities/health-worker-burnout/index.html

University of Otago, Wellington. (2023). *Movies for Undergraduate Public Health Teaching*. https://www.otago.ac.nz/wellington/departments/publichealth/undergraduate/movies-for-undergraduate-public-health-teaching

Walker, L. & Gorenstein, D. (2023). *She has Medicare and Medicaid. So Why Should It Take 18 Months to Get a Wheelchair?* National Public Radio. https://www.npr.org/sections/health-shots/2023/09/21/1200657834/she-has-medicare-and-medicaid-so-why-should-it-take-18-months-to-get-a-wheelchai

Woolf, S.H. (2023). Falling behind: The growing gap in life expectancy between the United States and other countries, 1933–2021. *American Journal of Public Health, 113*(9), 970–980. https://doi.org/10.2105/AJPH.2023.307310

Worldometer. (2023). *Life Expectancy of the World Population*. https://www.worldometers.info/demographics/life-expectancy/

Yphantides, N., Escoboza, S., & Macchione, N. (2015). Leadership in public health: New competencies for the future. *Frontiers in Public Health, 3*, 24. https://doi.org/10.3389/fpubh.2015.00024

Index

Note: **Bold** page numbers refer to tables and *italic* page numbers refer to figures.

Academy of Nutrition and Dietetics 192
accreditation 115
accuracy standards 72
advocacy 104–124; accomplishments
    through 117; advocate and 106; building
    consensus and promoting health policy
    118; challenges 121; coalition 111–112;
    communicating effectively 114–116;
    evaluation 122, **123**; funding 119;
    group 110; individual 107–110; *vs.*
    lobbying 104–105; opportunities 121–122;
    projects and staff management 117; raising
    awareness 118; relationships building
    116; role of 105–106; stakeholders and
    interested parties 110–111; systems and
    environmental change 119; task force 113;
    types 106–107; understanding health issue
    113–114; workgroup 112–113
Affordable Care Act (2010) 12, 14, 48, 185,
    188–189
Agency for Healthcare Research and Quality
    (AHRQ) 134, 185
agenda 153, 170
alcohol consumption 99
American Diabetes Association 83
American Evaluation Association (AEA)
    64, 75
American Journal of Health Promotion
    (journal) 164

American Journal of Public Health (journal)
    173
American Medical Association [AMA] 10
American Nurses Association 190
American Public Health Association (APHA)
    18, 108, 113, 164, 166, 173–174, 190
American School Health Association 175
American Society on Aging 175
Americans with Disabilities Act 109
Area Median Income (AMI) 119
Areas of Responsibility in HES 24–31, **25**,
    33, 45, 74; Advocacy 24, 28–29, 122;
    Assessment of Needs and Capacity 24–26,
    45; Communication 24, 29–30, 128;
    Ethics and Professionalism 24, 30–31, 169;
    Evaluation and Research 24, 27–28, 74;
    Implementation 24, 27, 85; Leadership and
    Management 24, 30, 144; Planning 24,
    26, 45
ask/advocacy ask 115, 121
Association of Prevention Teaching and
    Research 166
Association of Schools and Programs of
    Public Health 166
Association of Schools of Public Health
    (ASPH) 9
Association of State and Territorial Health
    Officials (ASTHO) 166, 186
Asthma Educator Specialist (AE-C) 166, 168

baseline data 43, 64
Behavioral Health Advisory Group 112
behavior change 68, 93, 97, 99, 130, 133, 138, 140, 152, 192
best practices 31, 43, 73, 75, 93, 106, 112, 115, 162–164, 167, 169, 170
bisphenol A (BPA) 118
Bloom's Taxonomy 170, *171*
brainstorming 56
Breast Cancer Awareness Month 139
budget 88–89; categories **90**

call for proposals 169
Campaign for Tobacco-Free Kids (CTFK) 191
Canadian Public Health Association (CPHA) 156
CDC Evaluation Planning Tools 72
CDC for program evaluation 69–71, *70*; conclusions justification 71; description 70; ensuring use and share lessons 71; evidence gathering 71; focus evaluation design 70–71; stakeholders engagement 70
CDC Foundation 182
CDC Health Communication Gateway website 135
CDC Office on Smoking and Health 131
CDC Tips from Former Smokers Campaign 130
Center for Community Health and Development 114
Centers for Disease Control and Prevention (CDC) 5, 13, 29, 45, 73, 91, 135, 136, 138, 140, 150, 181, 182, 185, 189, 191
Centers for Medicare and Medicaid (CMS) 185
Certified Diabetes Care and Education Specialist® (CDCES®) 166, 168
Certified Health Education Specialist (CHES®) 2, 11, 24, 31, 45, 85, 122, 128, 139, 144, 163, 166, 168; certification 34, 144, 162; credentials 172
Certified in Public Health (CPH) 166–168
challenges, in health advocacy 121; emerging topics 121; volunteer commitment *vs.* professional commitment 121
change management 151–153
CHES® exam 32–33; eligibility requirements 33; *vs.* MCHES® exam 33; test format 33–34
Children's Health Insurance Program 180
chronic disease management 4, 5
cigarette: advertisements 10; smoking 9–10, 40, 41
Closed Captions 139
coalition 84, 87, 111–112, 140
Coalition for National Health Education Organizations (CNHEO) 31

Code of Ethics for the Health Education Profession® (Code) 31–32, 172
Collective Impact Initiative 106
community: considerations for selecting model, framework/tool 54–55; definition 40
Community Action Plan 51, 52, 57
Community Context Assessment 50
community engagement 49, 82–83, 96; definition 82
Community Guide 93–94
community health 3; coalitions 84; data analysis 43; data sources 42–43; educators 2; specialists 2; status assessment 47–48
Community Health Assessment (CHA) 41, 44–45, 48, 51, 55, 58, 84, 86, 95, 100, 187; importance of 80–81
Community Health Assessment aNd Group Evaluation (CHANGE) 51–52, **52**, 54, 57
Community Health Dashboard 84
Community Health Improvement Plan (CHIP) 57, 81, 83, 84, 85, 95, 100, 111, 187
Community Health Needs Assessment *see* Community Health Assessment (CHA)
community health needs assessment and planning models 45–54; CHANGE 51–52, **52**; Forces of Change Assessment 47–49; MAPP 2.0 49, 49–50, *50*; Mobilizing for Action through Planning and Partnerships model 46–47, *47*; PRECEDE-PROCEED model *53*, 53–54
community hospitals 9
Community Partners Assessment 50
Community Preventive Services Task Force (CPSTF) 93, 130
Community Status Assessment 50
community themes and strengths assessment 47–49
Community Toolbox 55, 71
comorbidities 42
confidentiality 98, 145
consensus building 118
continual learning 162–163
Continuing Competency credits 172
continuing education 162, 172–175
continuing education contact hours (CECH) 172
costs: equipment 90; healthcare 5; indirect 90; match 90–91; materials and supplies 90; personnel 90; printing and marketing 90; revenue 91; travel 90
Council on Education for Public Health (CEPH) 168
COVID-19 pandemic 3, 5, 15, 29, 68, 112, 113, 129, 146, 147, 164, 167, 171, 181, 191, 193

CPH exam: domains 166–168, **167**; eligibility requirements for 168; test format 168
credibility 129, 139
Crip Camp: A disability revolution (documentary) 110
Crisis and Emergency Risk Communication (CERC) 136
cultural competency 133–136, 167
Culturally and Linguistically Appropriate Services (CLAS) 14, 75
culturally appropriate materials 134
culturally competent practices 75

de Beaumont Foundation 187
digital health technologies 195
direct-to-consumer pharmaceutical advertising (DTCPA) 10
domains in CPH exam 166–168, **167**; collaboration and partnership 167; communication 167; evidence-based approaches to public health 167; health equity and social justice 168; law and ethics 167; leadership 167; policy in public health 168; program management 168; program planning and evaluation 167; public health biology and human disease risk 167

education levels and health 92
electronic methods 128
elevator pitch/elevator speech 115, **116**
Emory Rollins School of Public Health 156
emotional appeal 138
employee health 3, 150
employee wellness programs 3
enabling factors 54
Endocrine Society 118
End the Backlog 119
environmental interventions 96
Environmental Protection Agency (EPA) 185
equipment costs 90
Essential Public Health Services (EPHS) 187, *187*
ethics, definition 30
European Food Safety Authority 118
evaluation phase 81, 83
evaluation report writing and dissemination 73–74; appendix with examples 73, 74; background and purpose 73; conclusion with recommendations 73, 74; describing evaluation methods 73; discussion of results 73–74; executive summary 73; results of evaluation 73
evaluation standards 72–73; accuracy standards 72–73; feasibility standards 72; propriety standards 72; utility standards 72
evidence-based interventions 43, 98
evidence-based recommendations 93, 94, 162, 165

Facebook 132
Fairfax County Community Health Improvement Plan (CHIP) 69, 74
feasibility standards 72
federal public health system **185**, 185–186
Food and Drug Administration (FDA) 118, 185
Forces of Change Assessment 47–49
formal advocacy 107
formative evaluation 67, 68
funding opportunity 4, 111

goal statements 86, **86**
Greek physicians 7
guaranteed income 112; programs 119
Guaranteed Income pilot program (2022) 119

health advocacy: challenges in 121; opportunities in 121–122
Health Affairs 182
health awareness campaign *see* health communication campaign
health behavior(s) 40, 41; theories 7
healthcare: costs 5; professionals 75; systems 188–190; in United States 184–185
health communication 96, 128–140; campaigns 130–132, 136, 137; components **129**, 129–130; cultural competency 133–136; evaluation 138; health literacy 133–136; oral and written skills utilized by HES 139; purpose 128–129; strategies for target audiences 133
health communication campaign 128–129
health communication channels 130–132; multimedia 130; print messages 131–132; public spaces and transit 131; social media and internet 132; telephone and cell phones 131; television and radio 130–131
health concerns 40, 43; limitations for 44, **44**
health dimensions 5–7; definitions 5, **6**; physical health 6; psychological health 6; social health 6; spiritual health 6
health disparities 11–12, 14, 75, 135, 136, 167, 195; definition 13; in health outcomes 15; types of 17
health education delivery, historical events in 7–11; academic preparation of health professionals in 20th century 8–9; ancient civilizations 7–8; Ottawa Charter 10, **11**; public health context in 20th century 9–10
health education practice 24
health education professionals 24
Health Education Specialist Practice Analysis II (2020) 24
Health Education Specialists (HES) 2, 180; Areas of Responsibility *see* Areas of Responsibility in HES; assessing communities 26; challenges in health

disparities 17–18; competencies and sub-competencies for 3, 24, 25, 31, 45, 74, 85, 122, 128, 144, 169; description 2; health dimensions and 5–7; improving health outcomes 40; job requirements 34, 35; NCHEC in 24; primary settings for 3–4; role of 96; workforce and projections 4–5

health equity 8, 13, 49, 75, 91, 98, 135, 136, 145, 167, 168, 184, 195

Health Impact Pyramid (HIP) 91, 91–93

health inequities 8, 14, 15, 50

health insurance 93, 136, 185, 188–189; access to affordable 14; marketplace 188; plans 188; premiums 3, 98; racial and ethnic disparities in 12

health literacy 96, 133–137, 167

health messages 128, 131, 133, 134

health needs 40–42, 44, 48, 50, 52, 84; identifying priorities 55–56

health outcomes 40–42, 43, 44, 46–48, 50, 62, 84, 105, 107, 135, 136, 190, 195

Health Promotion Practice (journal) 164

health status 13, 41, 47, 48; of United States 180–181

healthy behaviors 4, 6, 7, 62

Healthy Moms and Babies initiative 86, 87

healthy people: concept of 11; evolution of 13

Healthy People 2030 (HP 2030) 13, 43, 181

Healthy People: The Surgeon General's Report on Health Promotion and Disease Prevention 11

healthy weight 42

Hear Her campaign 132

high blood pressure 3, 184

Hispanic Paradox see Latino Paradox

Human Resources Department 109

Human Rights Campaign (HRC) 107

icebreakers 149

impact evaluation 67, 68

impact objectives 87

implementation of health education and promotion programs 191–193; limited resources 191; political influences 191–192; public health workforce 193; social media 192

implementation phase 88

income and health 92

indirect costs 90

individual/small group education type 96

indoor smoking bans 96, 99

infant mortality rates (IMR) 180, 181

infectious disease 4, 146, 186, 192, 195

influencers on social media 192

informal advocacy 106–107

informed consent 98

Instagram 132

Institute of Medicine Committee on Educating Public Health Professionals for the 21st Century (IOMCEPHP) 8, 9

intentionality 98, 149, 162, 163

internal evaluator vs. external evaluator 65, 65–66

Internal Revenue Services (IRS) 48; 501(C)(3) 48, 104–105

International Association of Providers of AIDS Care 175

intersectionality 17

interventions and programs 41, 44, 45, 49, 53, 56, 62–66; goals and objectives for 62, 63, 73, 74

invested partners and collaborators see stakeholders

Job Task Analysis 166

Johns Hopkins Bloomberg School of Public Health 104

Johns Hopkins University School of Hygiene and Public Health 9

Joint Committee on Standards for Educational Evaluation 72

Joyful Heart Foundation 119

Latino Paradox 184

leadership and management 144–158; definition 144; development 155, 155–156; job roles and opportunities 156–157, 157; qualities for 144–146, 145; skills to lead teams 146–151; skills to manage work 151–153

life expectancy 14, 181, 183

LinkedIn 157, 171

Live Healthy Miami Gardens 106

lobbying vs. advocacy 104–105

local public health system assessment 48

MAPP 2.0 46, 49, 49–50, 50

MAPP Handbook 55

Maryland Hospital Association (MHA) 112

mass media 99, 130, 140

Master Certified Health Education Specialist (MCHES®) 2, 11, 24, 31, 45, 85, 122, 128, 144, 163, 166, 168; certification 34, 144, 162; credentials 172

Master Settlement Agreement (MSA) 10

match costs 90–91

materials and supplies cost 90

Maternal, Infant, and Child Health Workgroup 181

maternal mortality rates (MMR) 180, 181

Mayors for a Guaranteed Income (MGI) 112

MCHES® exam 32–33; vs. CHES® exam 33; eligibility requirements 33; test format 33–34

Medicaid 180, 185, 188, 189

Medical Apartheid: The Dark History of Medical Experimentation on Black Americans from Colonial Times to the Present (Washington) 182
medical schools 9, 42
Medicare 180, 185, 188
mentor 30, 156, 173
Mind Tools 151
mission statement 85, **85**, 86
mobile apps 195
Mobilizing for Action through Planning and Partnerships model (MAPP) 46–47, **47**, 51, 54; community health status assessment 47–48; community themes and strengths assessment 47, 48; local public health system assessment 48
morbidity 42, 53
Move Your Way® campaign 162
multimedia campaigns 130
multiple evaluation methods 76
mutual respect 149

National Academy of Medicine *see* Institute of Medicine Committee on Educating Public Health Professionals for the 21st Century (IOMCEPHP)
National Action Plan to Improve Health Literacy 96, 136, 137
National Alliance on Mental Illness Virginia (NAMI) 109
National Association of Chronic Disease Directors 175
National Association of City and County Health Officials (NACCHO) 46, 49, 116, 150, 151, 166, 186
National Association of Diabetes Care and Education Specialists 175
National Board of Public Health Examiners (NBPHE) 166, 168
National Cancer Institute 131
National CLAS Standards 75, 95–96
National Collaborating Centre for Determinants of Health 17
National Collaborating Centre for Healthy Public Policy 17
National Commission for Health Education Credentialing, Inc. (NCHEC) 24, 25, 31, 32, 45, 156; role of 24
National Indian Health Board (NIHB) 115
National Institutes of Health (NIH) 135, 185
National Network of Public Health Institutes (NNPHI) 156
National Texting Portal 131
National Wellness Institute 5
The Nation's Health (newspaper) 164, 173
nominal group activity 56

objectives and action steps 57, 70, 81, 86
Office of the U.S. Surgeon General 6
Office on Minority Health 14
onboarding 147, 164
opportunities, in health advocacy 121–122; engaging members of community 121–122; network of support 122
optimal health 6, 18, 187
Ottawa Charter 10, **11**
Our Epidemic of Loneliness and Isolation 6
outcome evaluation 67, 68
outcome objectives 87

Partnership for a Healthier Fairfax (PFHF) 84
Patient Education Assessment Tool 134
Patient Protection and Affordable Care Act (2010) 14
people management 117
performance reviews 148
personnel costs 90
Physical Activity Guidelines for Americans 162
Physical Activity. The Arthritis Pain Reliever campaign 138
physical health 6
PLACES tool 182, 183
planning and implementation of interventions and programs: additional planning groups 83–84; benefits and barriers 96–99; community engagement 82–83; Community Guide 93–94; Health Impact Pyramid *91*, 92–93; importance of needs assessments 80–81; levels of prevention 94–95, **95**; new and existing 95–96; in schools 98; selecting and developing 91–92; steps in *see* program planning; tools 85–91; types 96, **97**; in workplaces 98
Planning Committee 81–83
planning phase 80
policy-level intervention 96, 122
practice analysis study 24
PRECEDE-PROCEED Model *53*, 53–54
predisposing factors 54
pre-planning phase 81, 86
Prevention and Public Health Fund 191
primary healthcare providers (PCPs) 188
primary prevention activities 94, 95
printed materials 128
printing and marketing costs 90
privacy 98
process evaluation 67, 68
process objectives 86–87
professional development funds 164
professional development plan 163
professional development strategies for HES 161–175; Certified in Public Health 166–168; continual learning 162–163; contributing to public health field 169–172; current events 165; developing and refining

skills 165–166; literature 164; maintaining CHES and MCHES credentials 172; participating in conferences and workshops 163–164; professional organizations 172–174; specialized professional organizations 174–175, **175**

professional newsletters 164–165

professional staff 121

program evaluation process 62; CDC framework for 69–71; conducting 65–67; planning 64–65; practices and strategies for success 75–76; purpose 62–64, **63**; report writing and dissemination 73–74; standards 72–73; types **67**, 67–69

program planning 81, **82**; choosing and/or developing interventions 81; developing goals, objectives, and action items 81; evaluation 81; implementation 81; pre-planning 81

project management 27, 152

Project Management Institute (PMI) 152

Project Management Professional (PMP®) 152

propriety standards 72

psychological health 6

public health (PH) 6, 44, 104; accreditation 115; campaigns 3, 135; context in 20th century 9–10; education in 190; educators 9; nursing 190; profession 2; schools 9; systems 48, 104; workforce 180

Public Health Accreditation Board 151

Public Health Advocacy Newsletters 165

Public Health Diabetes Newsletters 165

Public Health Foundation 155

Public Health Institute Center for Health Leadership & Impact 155

public health interventions, opportunities for 194–196; foundation of success 195; leveraging technology 195; return on investment (ROI) promotion 196; working towards health equity 195

Public Health Media Library 138

Public Health National Center for Innovations (PHNCI) 187

Public Health Newsletters 165

public health professionals 2, 4, 99, 129, 135, 136, 145–146, 180; academic preparation in 20th century 8–9

public health systems in United States 184–185

Public Health Workforce Interests and Needs Survey 193

Public Health Workforce Resilience Resource Library 150

Public Information Officer (PIO) 136

qualitative data 42, 43, 50

quality of healthcare 12, 75; racial and ethnic minorities in 12

quality of life 5, 30, 42, 53, 94, 96

quantitative data 42, 43, 47, 50

racism 135; definition 12

rape test kits 119

Real Cost campaign 196

refinement process, in health messages 133

reinforcing factors 54

Request for Proposals (RFP) 119

return on investment (ROI) 196

revenue costs 91

Robert's Rules of Order 153

Robert Wood Johnson Foundation 182

Rockefeller Foundation 9

Rockefeller Sanitary Commission 8

root causes 114, 119, 195

Rural Health Information Hub 146, 193

Rural Health Promotion and Disease Prevention Toolkit 193

Safe Routes to School 92

Sandy Hook Promise *Start with Hello* curriculum 98

secondary prevention activities 94, 95

self-assessment 148

Sexual Assault Kit Initiative 119

sign-on letters 108–109

skills for leading teams: performance reviews 148; relationships with community members 150–151; supervision 147–148; supporting team members 149–150; team building 149

skills to manage work 151–157; change management 152–153; meeting facilitation 153–154, *154*; project management 152; strategic planning 151

SmokefreeTXT program 131

Smoking and Health: Report of the Advisory Committee to the Surgeon General 9–10

social determinants of health (SDOH) 13–17, **14**, 29, 42, 44, 50, 92, 93, 135, 136, 180, 182–184

social-ecological model 99, **99**

social health 6

social justice 14, 144, 145, 168

social media 128, 130, 132, 139, 192, 195

Social Security Act (1935) 9

Society for Human Resource Management 148

Society for Public Health Education (SOPHE) 110, 174

Society of Health and Physical Educators 175

South Carolina Department of Health and Environmental Control (SCDHEC) 112

Special Primary Interest Groups 173

Specific, Measurable, Attainable, Realistic, and Time-bound (SMART) objectives **87**, 87–88

spiritual health 6
stakeholders 45, 46, 70, 110, 112; and interested party analysis matrix 111
state and local public health system 186–187
Steering Committee 83, 84
strategic planning 30, 46, 105, 151, 187
streaming services 131
stress management 3, 9, 40
structural racism 184
Structural Racism and Discrimination (SRD) 183–184
subject matter experts (SME) 24, 31, 83, 114, 121, 122, 166
Substance Abuse and Mental Health Administration (SAMHSA) 185
summative evaluation 67, 69
supervision 147–148
system-level intervention 122
systems change 119
systems problems 189

tailored messages 96, 133
tailoring 8, 133
talking point 28, 114–115
target audience 129, 136; segmentation 133
target population 65, 70, 73, 74, 76, 83, 93, 98
task force 24, 29, 30, 83, 84, 110, 113
team building 146, 149
team culture 149
telehealth platforms 195
tertiary prevention activities 94, 95
Text4Baby program 97
text messages/messaging 96, 97, 131
Thinking in Systems (TiS).approach 189–190
TikTok 132
timeline 54, 66, 71, 74, 81, 85, 88, 89, 151, 154, 168
tobacco cessation tools 99
tobacco control campaigns 99
Tobacco Control Coalition 84
tobacco prevention programs 99
tobacco products 9, 40, 41, 99
tools4dev organization 110
TRAIN online learning platform 155
Trauma-Informed Community Network 84
travel costs 90

Tribal Public Health Departments 115
trust 30, 45, 105, 116, 133, 145, 149, 151, 159, 163, 180, 191
Trust for America's Health (The Trust) 191

underinsured people 188
Understanding and Preventing Burnout among Public Health Workers: Guidance for Public Health Leaders 150
Unequal Treatment: Confronting Racial and Ethnic Disparities in Health Care 12
unhealthy behavior 62, 128
uninsured people 188
United Nations Population Division 181
University of Otago, Wellington 194
University of Wisconsin 5
Unnatural Causes: Is inequality making us sick? (documentary series) 10, 184
U.S. Bureau of Labor Statistics (BLS) 2, 4
U.S. Department of Health and Human Services (HHS) 11, 93, 96, 185, 186
U.S. Department of Health and Human Services and Office of Minority Health 75
U.S. Surgeon General 9, 11
utility standards 72

vision statement 85, **85**, 86
volunteer commitment *vs.* professional commitment 121
volunteers 121, 122, 147–148
voting 55, 56, 104, 153

wearable devices 195
White House Executive Order 13995 (2021) 113
WHO Commission on Social Determinants of Health 14, 15
Who Will Keep the Public Healthy? Educating Public Health Professionals for the 21st Century 8
Wild to Mild campaign 140
windshield tours 42
Women, Infants and Children (WIC) 196
workforce diversity 98
work plan 74, 85, 88, *89*, 100, 151, 168
World Health Organization (WHO) 5, 13, 17
Worldometer 181

For Product Safety Concerns and Information please contact our
EU representative GPSR@taylorandfrancis.com Taylor & Francis
Verlag GmbH, Kaufingerstraße 24, 80331 München, Germany